Sit With It:
The Truth Behind Weight loss

Sit With It:
The Truth Behind Weight loss

ANDERS GRANT, MS, RD, LDN

To order additional copies of this book, contact:
Xlibris Corporation
1-888-795-4274
www.Xlibris.com
Orders@Xlibris.com
36548

Acknowledgment

Thanks to my children, my sisters and friends for their loving support and encouragement. A special thanks to the artists Richard Monroe and Steven in Tennessee, for their flexibility and ability to see what I see.

Preface

If you have battled with *dieting*, have tried more than a few diets or have lost weight and regained it, this book is for you. This book represents possibly the last book you will need on your weight loss journey. However, you must be *coachable* (willing to be guided and instructed) to go through the weight loss process. You must also be willing to discard everything you think you know as you actively go through each step of this book. *Sit-With-It: The Truth Behind Weight Loss* is ideally for those who are ready for change. It is for those who are ready to commit to eating healthy and increasing their level of physical activity. These lifestyle changes must be as vital and important to you as getting up each day and going to work or taking care of your family. If you are not really ready and are just looking at another way to start something and then give up, this book is not for you. You will be guided through the weight loss steps using the *sit-with-it* process. You will be able to lose weight and maintain the weight loss. It is a process which takes time, but it works.

Unfortunately, there are no quick fixes (e.g., magic pills, patches or wands). To lose the weight and keep it off requires constant vigilance, as well as, healthy lifestyle changes. It also requires an increase in your current level of physical activity and a commitment to loving and taking care of yourself. It is my hope that by the end of reading this book, you will be able to do all of the above.

As you read you should notice your movement through the behavior modification stages of change, as developed by Prochaska, DiClemente, and Norcross. You will be assisted in adopting new and healthy behavior habits as developed by Maxie C. Maultsby, Jr., M.D., a pioneer of Rational Behavior Therapy (RBT).

As you go through the processes of behavior change, you will begin to identify the possible psychosocial dynamics behind weight gain and weight loss and you will find solutions unique to your situation. Are you ready? Are you tired of the endless yo-yo weight on, weight off? If so, read on to stop believing the lies and paying the high costs attached to sickness and disease: not to mention the toll it takes on your self-respect, self-love, self-esteem and quality of life.

We begin with the basics of good nutrition, review the energy equation, dispel some myths, and give you the tools to take off the weight and keep it off. You are encouraged to look deeper inside your beautiful self and attempt to understand in your own way that weight gain is not just about food. It is the relationship you have formed with food and the power you have turned over to it. Finally, you will acquire the strategies and skills to keep you in weight maintenance, once your weight loss goals have been realized.

Be prepared to allow yourself to be coached through the process. Go beyond the comfortable and experience the uncomfortable. If a negative response is triggered, you are encouraged to explore it objectively and without judgment. Remember, when the student is ready, the teacher shows up.

Consider the best way to start is to begin. However, before turning the next page to begin your journey, ask yourself this question: "Is being healthy the wisest way for me to live?" If you respond, "yes," then read on.

Note: 1) If you have a diagnosed medical condition (e.g., diabetes, renal failure or mental illness), please consult with your physician, therapist and/or registered dietitian before making dietary changes.
2) For confidentiality purposes, the names of individuals used in examples have been changed to preserve their privacy.

Introduction

Weight loss is a very personal thing. Most people feel threatened and exposed. Their greatest fear is they will be seen as failures. This is why they will try to find something wrong with reading this book. If you doubt this, think about the many diets you have tried. Now look at the many changes to the "diet" you made before ever trying it (e.g., "I will eat breakfast and lunch, but not the dinner," or "I do not need the snack."). You modified it to meet your tastes.

This is why one of the first challenges to weight loss is acknowledging you do not know everything and in this case, you are NOT the expert. Accept the "diet" did not work because *YOU* changed it from its original design, or you did not follow it to the letter, or you stopped doing it.

The second challenge is to accept you are wrong, and have been for a while. You have been wrong about whether or not you can lose weight. You can lose weight, but you may be having difficulty understanding that the excess weight is a symbol of something else. You have not maintained the lost weight because you have not dealt with the *something else*. For example, most people like to believe they are right most of the time. So as they try to lose weight without accepting it is okay to not know it all, or it is okay to be wrong, they join a weight loss program and only listen to the parts they want to hear. As they listen to how it works, they question it and make edits to how they think it is going to work for them. They even personalize it to how they think it will work. Then, when changes are not seen quickly enough or at all, they blame the weight loss program.

Halt! Give up wanting to be right, because here is where you will get your greatest insight. Listen. Here is someone telling you what to do to be successful in something you think you want. However, you continue listening to your own familiar, fearful voice saying "I can't." So, before the program even begins, you have already decided you are going to prove yourself right with, "I can't." Also, note your inner self saying, "This will not last long," and "I will not be able to keep it off"—even as you are losing weight.

My hope therefore, is for you to realize the greatest potential at its source—your mind. The *sit-with-it* process works. You have to trust it will work and you are being provided with sound and loving guidance. There is no judgment here. You start by giving up the right to think you know how best to lose weight. If you start with purity—a clean slate—you will avoid getting stuck in your old ruts. See this as a journey without obstacles or barriers (e.g., I have no time or I am too busy). Recognize the importance of making a change, because being in old ruts has contributed to your weight gain. It is in your best interest to drop your wall of defenses so you can see results quickly and more permanently.

Chapter 1

The Lord is my Shepherd; I shall not want.

(Psalm 23:1)

Good nutrition

To first understand good nutrition, it is important to believe the world has an abundant supply of food. If you wanted, you could even grow what you needed. You do not have to believe the lie of, "I will starve if I miss a meal." First of all, you will not starve if you miss a meal. You may get hungry, but you will not *starve*. Here is where it all begins. We tell ourselves lies, rationalize them, and then believe them. The outcome is to temporarily overindulge in an extra serving of something. These indulgences bring consequences— guilt, shame, feeling bad, maybe even sickness or diseases.

We go to all-you-can-eat buffets and fill ourselves far beyond a comfort level. The paradox is you are not cheating the business owner, you are only cheating yourself! You are the one gaining weight and thereby increasing your risk factors for certain diseases. In the end, it will be you paying for more than you bargained for.

The food supply is dwindling

When we overeat, we may believe the food supply is going to run out, and therefore, we have to have it all NOW. We have to eat all we can in this moment. Is this a familiar scene? You see it is late and you know you are about to go to bed. You have not eaten all day, so you tell yourself, "I have to eat something." Again, STOP! You do not have to eat something. What you probably have to do is to go to bed. You will be fine when you get up the next morning. You will still be alive! (Remember, if you have a medical diagnosis of diabetes, or are on special medicines, please consult your physician and/or registered dietitian for further nutritional recommendations.) In a practical way, if you are telling yourself the food supply is going to be finished, or you are going to starve, you will be more likely to eat something; despite the fact your body does not need it. This is part of the psychological (self-talk) cycle which has to be reconnected to rational thinking. Instead, say to yourself, "Yes, I am tired and hungry, but I do not need to eat right now. I will go to bed now, and tomorrow I will eat an enjoyable breakfast." (Refer to example in Chapter 6).

Being deprived is awful

We walk around believing being deprived is awful. Who told us so? Why do we have a negative connotation about being deprived? Yes, to be deprived of basic needs may be uncomfortable, but the truth is being overindulgent is what is really happening. On a subconscious level we may be feeling we have been stuffing down feelings (e.g., held back a comment to a rude co-worker, been overlooked for a promotion, or pretended everything is okay with others). Now, when it comes to eating, we are going to do what we want: we worked hard today, or we deserve it. It is the only thing we feel we have control over or a right to. Hence, we call food our comfort. Now, start to realize food comforted you because it filled an emotional, psychological, or physical void and allowed you to go into a state of *avoidance*. It was not because you were physically *starved*.

Behavior stages of change

Stages of change are stages an individual may go through before actually making a behavior change. You are probably at one of the stages proposed by Prochaska, et al.

Pre-contemplative stage of change: you are not accepting or personalizing the problem and therefore, are unable to recognize the need for change.

Contemplative stage of change: you are thinking about change but have not really decided yet how to effect the change.

Preparation stage of change: you have started to develop a plan (probably thinking of joining a gym or buying exercise equipment).

Action stage of change: you have taken steps to change and are modifying behaviors.

Maintenance stage of change: you have acquired skills and support for continued change and are consistently following through for more than six weeks. Reinforcement and encouragement are required at this stage. This really could be *key*!

Relapse stage of change: is the final stage and you may need renewed commitment and motivation as a result of having either lost interest and motivation, have been overwhelmed by what the changes have cost you personally (e.g., interrelationships with others), or you may have become disheartened.

Which stage are you in?

Commitment re-defined

The commitment we are talking about here is one of being honest and truthful: not just with yourself but with those with whom you are in a relationship. Through the *sit-with-it* process, you will be required to commit to certain strategies, goals and relationships. Not holding your commitment to those relationships may cost you the ultimate prize of redefining who you chose to be as a human being. In essence, you will come to understand what you are committed to and you will keep your word. You will follow through with what you say you are going to do: it is your agreement with yourself to honor your word.

Take the challenge

Life is a process and we should be moving forward with it: move to a higher level. All change takes effort and desire (Sue Patton Thoele). Change is not always easy, but once you make yourself face your tiger and overcome the fear, the rewards you glean are untouchable. I liken the experience to when I ran my first 100-mile race. As I was on my journey, I kept focused on my commitment to finish. It was not until two weeks after the race (after the pain and discomfort dissipated), that I actually experienced the victory of it! I had done it! I had set a goal, trained for, and accomplished it against extreme odds. Standing on the mountain top of accomplishment, this eagle's wings could not be clipped!

Sitting-with-it is no different. It is the final stage of weight loss where you go through the process using the skills outlined and always recall your goal to be your commitment. You set a goal (weight loss), train (practice *sitting-with-it*) and arrive on the mountain top of accomplishment (celebrating the new you). Yes, change is not always easy because it is uncomfortable. Hang in there and you will achieve the rewards of your life-changing efforts.

Fundamentals and cautions

There are some individuals, who because of metabolic disturbances caused by hormones or medications, are challenged with regard to losing weight. This should not be used as an excuse. Your physician is the best one to make a diagnosis after running appropriate tests. He or she can make recommendations which can help you to lose weight despite these challenges. A vast majority of people are able to lose weight with the guidance of a health care team experienced in helping individuals with weight loss. However, for those with only a few pounds to lose (less than 30 pounds), a healthcare team may or may not be necessary—you, along with the help and supervision of your physician, will have to decide.

A balanced health care team usually consists of a registered dietitian, physician, counselor or therapist, and perhaps a personal trainer. There are multiple modalities of weight loss treatment such as pharmacotherapy, surgery, low-calorie diets, very low calorie diets, increasing physical activity level, behavior modification techniques/strategies, nutrition education, counseling or hypnosis.

These modalities may be used singly or in combination. For example, pharmacotherapy and a low calorie diet may work for one individual depending on where the client is after the initial assessment. The client later may change to a low calorie diet with increased physical activity to reach the next stage of weight loss or maintenance. The approach or modality used will be determined by your health care team and will be modified to meet your changing needs over time. The continued support and encouragement from a therapist or counselor and/or support group will also be beneficial.

If you are interested in losing weight, first seek medical clearance from your physician because a lot of weight loss' efficacy relies on your involvement in moderate to intense level exercises for durations of up to 30 minutes (and, depending on your goals, 60-90 minutes). Also, with your physician involved in your commitment to take off those extra pounds, she will be better able to manage you medically in the event medicines are indicated for use or change in the initial treatment and/or maintenance phase.

The role/credentials of a registered dietitian

How can a registered dietitian help? A registered dietitian is someone who has earned an undergraduate or graduate degree (in the field of food and nutrition from an accredited college or university), then interned in a 900-hour six to 24-month, supervised, didactic program and is Board certified. Staying abreast of updates and changes in the field is mandatory and accomplished through meeting continuing education requirements. Meeting these requirements is a condition of maintaining licensure. They keep current in nutrition specialty fields such as weight loss, food science and technology, gerontology, pediatrics, diabetes self-management, nutrition support, eating disorders or sports nutrition. Further, a registered dietitian has an extensive background in the sciences including nutrition science, physiology, biochemistry, organic chemistry, microbiology, economics, statistics, sociology and computer science. They are qualified to work in a number of different industries such as food product and design, quality assurance, sales, advertising, healthcare, education, community or hospitality.

The assistance of a registered dietitian is important because a complete nutritional assessment can be performed to assess a broad range of issues such as overall risk status, Body Mass Index (BMI), motivation to lose weight, self-efficacy, stage of behavioral change, previous weight loss attempts and outcomes, environmental factors, goals, and obstacles to weight loss.

Basics of weight loss

The basic premise of weight loss is the equation: energy in = energy out. For example, if you normally consume 2,000 calories and you expend 2,000 calories, you break even; there is no weight gain or weight loss, only weight maintenance. However, if you consume 1500 calories and expend 2,000 calories you will have weight loss, because you did not provide enough energy for your body to run on and therefore it had to go to fat stores to use for energy. The converse is also true, if you consume 2,000 calories and expend 1500 calories, you will have weight gain, because you took in more energy in the form of food, which now gets converted and stored as body fat (adipose tissue). 3500 extra calories = 1 pound body fat. Therefore, for most, a reduction of 500 calories/day will equal one pound weight loss per week (or minus 250 calories/d = 1 pound weight loss/2 weeks).

So, looking at the law of averages, you can see if you consistently eat more than you spend, you will continue to have weight gain. The key here is consistently. As we age, we expend less energy. Therefore, if our eating habits do not change, it is easy to see how weight gain occurs.

There will be times when you eat less and times when you eat more. But if the times you eat more far outweigh the times you eat less, you will have weight gain. I have had clients who reported eating less than 500 calories per day Monday to Friday, but then consuming greater than 3,000 calories per day on the other two days. This flawed mythical strategy will definitely not lead to weight loss. Why? Because you will be teaching your body to starve Monday to Friday, and this puts it into conservation-mode, causing it to need less than the usual caloric requirements and you start to burn less energy—much like a bear going into hibernation.

Common weight loss excuses

I hear a lot of my clients saying things like: "I can't lose weight;" "I have tried all the diets," (as they hand me a list of five or more they have tried); "Just tell me what to eat;" "I do not have time to exercise;" "I do not have time to plan a meal;" "I get home too late;" "I work odd hours;" "I am on the road a lot;" "Everyone in my family looks like me;" "I have been big all my life;" "I have thyroid problems;" or "I shake when I do not eat." The excuses are numerous. Please recognize they are mostly excuses and can be ruled out with a complete physical exam by your physician.

In all my years of teaching weight loss, the energy equation has not changed, and therefore, weight loss can mainly be achieved by changing some aspect of your lifestyle. The initial step would be to acknowledge you might be afraid of change and start there. The initial work is not about food, but in discovering the relationships around food and how you use it as a coping strategy. You may even find you are not ready for change—and this too is okay.

Too many times as dietitians, we find ourselves spending more time establishing our credentials and defending our recommendations than in making headway to effect change. In part, this is due to fad diets and nutrition myths. It seems everyone would like to believe he is the expert when it comes to food; possibly because of erroneously equating nutrition with cooking. Also, because dietitians specialize in food, a misperception is we are cooks, food service workers or caterers. The field of food and nutrition is a science and weight loss is really a numbers game. Change is possible when you are willing to recognize your excuses/stories and choose to change your beliefs, thoughts, and behaviors (in that order).

The complications of food and its basic chemical components are not so readily visible to even the most seasoned "cooks." In fact, if you ask someone who has been baking for years, "What is in your apple pie recipe?" they respond, "Oh, I just put a bit of this and that" without giving the specifics (1 cup, ½ teaspoon, etc.) because it has become rote, and they feel that to anyone else talking about food, it is obvious! However, the science of food is far different from the art of cooking, as it regards proper nutrition and weight loss. For example, there have been lots of talk about what the best composition of a meal should be (i.e., fats vs. carbohydrates vs. protein percentages), without taking into account the bottom line: calories in = calories out. Yes, there are exceptions as with sports or support nutrition, but we are talking about the average dieter here, so do not become distracted.

Our bodies are specially and intricately designed. This is not to say, however, there are not times when one can consume too few calories and not see the intended weight loss. In such a situation, however, if that behavior is maintained over an extended period of time, even the staunchest weight loss participant will see weight loss. The average dieter, however, is described as an individual who jumps from diet to diet in hopes they will land on one that will produce a quick fix. The fact is it took many years to accumulate the excess weight and it will take time to lose it.

The subtotal of things*

The truth about weight loss is there are no quick fixes. Even bariatric surgeries are not quick fixes. For some, they are temporary fixes. They can be desperate measures that usually are the last resort for some and the beginning of misery for others. In summary:

When ENERGY IN = ENERGY OUT, there is weight maintenance.

When ENERGY IN > ENERGY OUT, there is weight gain.

When ENERGY IN < ENERGY OUT, there is weight loss.

---

*   Note previous exceptions.

Chapter 2

Could it be . . . ?

Hummm?

Could it be the rise in obesity is related to a sense of dissatisfaction in people's lives; therefore, when they call food their comfort, it is real? It is their only comfort. If so, obesity could represent the dissatisfaction with their lives in the choices they have made. For example, people, who are not happy with the career they chose or the job situation in which they find themselves (i.e., did not finish school or got too much schooling), may not want to take ownership for their choices. They then cast the blame onto food, and eating becomes their scapegoat. They eat away their pain and grief for the future for which they hoped and which will never be realized. Maybe they do not feel equipped to meet the future head-on.

Do you realize that obesity, cigarette smoking, sexually-transmitted diseases, as well as other negative risk factors can truncate your life? Yet, despite all the education, there is still a rise in these diseases/instances. The sad part is you have a choice and a voice. You can take a stand for something. You can choose to make changes. But first, you must start to believe change is both necessary and possible. To do this, we look at your core beliefs. Whatever you believe in your core—in your center, your visceral area—is what you will act out.

What does it mean to lose weight?

Once the weight is lost, the battle is not over. You really have to look at and work on totally accepting and loving yourself. I have seen too many people lose weight only to regain it (and sometimes more). Weight loss maintenance requires constant vigilance. Being part of a loving and supportive structure is vitally important in discovering for you what life experiences and perceptions contributed to your weight gain. As mentioned earlier, weight loss is not just about food. At times it can be about power and control, fear and loss. It is worth doing the research. For some of you, reading this book and other books may be enough. For others, getting into counseling, whether individual or group, may be what is needed. Whatever you decide, start by entering into the *sit-with-it* process.

A particular client comes to mind when I talk about entering the *sit-with-it* process. For privacy purposes we will call her Julie. When Julie initially came to me, she was in a "ball of denial." She resisted most of my recommendations and suggestions, until weeks later, she was able to identify eating was her coping strategy. She would appear to solicit my help, but she was always changing this subject. In conversation with her, you would find her talking about things other than the impact her eating behaviors were having on her life. She was therefore not attached to the conversation. When she ate, she was also not attached to the act of eating, and this easily set her up for overeating; as she was never present to what she was doing in the here and now. She was, psychologically, somewhere else and was not the one eating. So when she said, "I do not eat anything" she was telling the truth as it appeared to her. The reason she developed this coping mechanism, would be best addressed by a therapist or counselor.

Start to identify the challenges to your weight loss

A possible challenge to weight loss is that you are not willing to give up something. I am referring to giving up the argument of having too many controls on your life (like paying taxes, stopping at red lights, going the posted speed limit, balancing your check book, taking care of your kids or family or going to work). I invite you to give up the freedom of arguing against taking control of one more thing in your life—your eating behaviors. Recognize being overweight is being out of control. To stick to a diet or meal plan, to make the commitment necessary to have weight loss, requires digging your heels in and taking control of a situation that has gotten out of control. Therefore, if you feel like your life is out of control, how could you possibly control your eating habits? To do so would be in direct contradiction to how you were feeling about your life. All this under the façade, "I have it all together."

If this is beginning to sound very confusing, hang in there, because by being overweight you reinforce, in fact, your life is out of control. This is all part of your story. I hope you are beginning to see just how we create our own confusion, and then expect to make sense out of losing weight. No wonder we travel from diet to diet—it helps to keep the confusion going. Think about it, would it be any fun to start a diet and actually live with the results of keeping the weight off? "Yes," you say? No, because if that were the truth for you, you would do it. But you do not. In reality, you see the results and then go back to your old way of doing things and say, "The diet did not work." The funny thing is, everyone agrees with you! Why? Because, they too have all done it at one time or another—tried something that worked, stopped doing it, and said it was not for them. No, you are not crazy, but you are beginning to awake from your slumber if it all seems futile for you. Keep reading.

When people ask me to give them a *diet* they ask, "Will I feel hungry?" "Will I feel full?" Why are you asking me this? If going on a diet means you will be eating less, what is your real question? Pause. Exhale. Take the time to stop and look at what is going on for you psychologically, environmentally, socially, emotionally, physically, and financially that could be causing feelings of hunger.

For example, in an attempt to identify possible sources of *hunger* start in the bedroom. If your sex life is such that both partners are equally content with the arrangement, or if you or your partner do not have a negative body image, or negative image of his/her sexuality, then turn to the family room. Are there unresolved relationship issues? Is there dissension between you and a family member, friends, co-workers, or neighbors? Are there situations in which you are now taking care of an adult parent and there is some anger, resentment or blame? If there are no issues there, then look at your career. Do you have job satisfaction? Do you like your boss, co-workers or work? If there are no issues there, then look at your education. Have you met your educational goals? Are you being frustrated in your attempts to coerce others to complete their education? If there are no issues there, look at your finances. Are you earning the type of income you feel you should be earning at your current level of expenses, experience and education? Are you spending more than you make? Are you in debt? Do you gamble? Do you shop excessively?

The list of questions is inexhaustible. However, the questions above delve into areas where *hunger* is generated. These are vulnerable areas that can create an emotional void. Until these areas are identified, explored, dealt with, worked out, and resolved, weight loss or its maintenance may not be realized. If in all this chaos weight loss is realized, then weight maintenance may continue to be elusive. When you are eating past the point of satiety, there is clearly an underlying issue. If you have been classified as Overweight, or Class I-III Obese, or you have health issues, or familial or relationship issues directly related to being overweight, I would challenge you to look at the root of those hunger pangs more closely. Fish out what they actually are and deal with them. Then, just *SIT-WITH-IT* (explained in Chapter 4).

At this point, you should be in the *pre-contemplative stage* of change.

Chapter 3

He shall die without instruction;
and in the greatness of his folly he shall go astray.
(Prov. 5:23)

Getting started

The most challenging stage of weight loss is getting started because you are being asked to change and change usually triggers a certain level of anxiety and fear—especially if you do not feel good about yourself.

The saboteur is in us all. It appears as negative self-talk, rationalizations and excuses telling you why you should not start or to put it off till later. You will hear yourself saying, "I will start tomorrow." "I will start after my vacation or wedding." "I will wait until . . ." You will be assaulted with a multitude of thought processes aimed at your not staying committed to your new healthy living and fitness goals. Do not fight the thoughts; just become aware of them. Become aware of the conversations you have with yourself that lead you to the behaviors you choose.

Behavior theories attempt to explain why we humans do what we do. It attempts to explain how behavior is learned from the environment based on one's response to it. Following the example given in Chapter 5, you will see how Rational Behavior Therapy (RBT), can help those same individuals, as it attempts to help people identify their core belief(s).

Using RBT, you may identify one of your core belief is that, "In order to be accepted, I have to be a people-pleaser," and how you act out with food enables you to identify this belief. I am sure you have heard, "The way to a man's heart is through his stomach." So, depending on your role as the nurturer and/or provider, you behave in a certain manner. For example, as a nurturer, you feed your family and as a provider you tell yourself that your family has to eat—that is how you measure your success.

Here is how it works: a husband and wife contribute to the perpetuation of the false belief that food is a comfort. They then pass on this myth to their family in their behaviors of making food the focal point of holidays and patting their bellies after a good, hearty meal where, although uncomfortable, they can still make room for more.

Can you identify with this? How many times have you complimented the chef/cook with a deep sigh of contentment and satisfaction looking like a Cheshire cat with cream still on its whiskers?

My oldest daughter told me that she was able to identify when she started to overeat by a very innocent event. While at a friend's home she was offered a full packet (2 servings) of Ramen Noodles. Until that point, she had only eaten half a pack because she did not *believe* she could eat more than that. However, the sister prepared a whole pack for each of them and she ate it. She then continued to rationalize overeating and kept testing her limits. Using RBT, she was able to make this identification (three years and with a 20 pound weight gain after the fact), and she was able to choose to only consume "half a pack" and her continued weight gain stopped.

Paradoxically when you look at how we acquire a taste for certain foods and beverages, it is quite comical. In fact, our body initially rejects it, but we override its initial response, and over time, we began to actually enjoy certain items and at times, overindulge in them.

Just stop and think about the first time you drank coffee, beer, wine or ate yogurt. You pulled back from the taste. But, after telling yourself it was "okay," you went on to develop "a taste for it."

Is it any wonder we are overweight? We have historically overridden our body's internal "gag" signal in order to acquire a certain taste. It is time to retrieve our *gag* signal and get back to the basics of respecting our instincts and honoring our soul.

At this point, you should be at the *contemplative stage* of change.

Chapter 4

If thou be wise, thou shalt be wise for thyself . . .
(Proverb 9:12)

What it means to SIT-WITH-IT

To *sit-with-it* requires your attention to your psycho-spiritual connection. Explore it. This connection lies between the will of wanting to lose weight and calling on your Higher Power to help you stay on track. It seems that we are more able to commit to a Higher Power than to ourselves. Therefore, this bond is crucial to establish.

The realization that we are one with the universe and, therefore what we do with our bodies is part of the mosaic of our destiny, makes it clearer that taking care of our bodies is not an option. Rather it is a spiritual and physical requirement if we want to continue to enjoy a healthy existence. Start by settling down in a quiet place where you feel safe and free. You may want to wear headphones and listen to soothing sounds, either sitting up or lying down. Allow your mind to wonder to a beautiful place with refreshing sights, sounds, smells and tastes. Recognize that each beautiful sensation means each of your internal organs is bathing in a sea of love, forgiveness and kindness. Experience this as self-love and commit to *bathing* your body with good nutrition and increased physical activity. Then, as you engage in your ritual of eating and exercising, be present to what your body is telling you and honor its *full* signal.

Therefore, to *sit-with-It,* means that you take time to PAUSE. You contemplate the consequences of forgoing your goals to overall good health and fitness. It means recalling to your memory the goals and the strategies you pre-planned to help you in your weakest moments. It means you *pause* to take the time to recall how good you felt the last time you accomplished a goal. You will have to *sit-with-it,* each time you think of "giving in to your cravings," despite your goals. Over time, your need to *sit-with-it* diminishes because your new habits will have replaced the old habits and desires. Foods you thought you could not live without before are no longer a temptation. Old patterns of behavior will change and you will find that you are able to adapt to a new chosen attitude more easily. You will be able to experience the power and control you have always desired. It requires work—but it is possible and worthwhile.

Stage 1 of sit-with-it (recognize)

SIT-WITH-IT is a state of mind.

SIT-WITH-IT brings into focus your commitment to change.

SIT-WITH-IT refutes the irrational thoughts and excuse-making that plague us and cause relapse.

SIT-WITH-IT recalls the feelings of success when you followed through on your commitment.

SIT-WITH-IT means to keep your eyes on the ball—your goal.

SIT-WITH-IT means to re-direct your attention away from food.

In the past, food served as a distraction. Now you will go through experiencing your thoughts/emotions and come out on the other side. Hopefully you will no longer avoid your feelings or thoughts because to do so, will cost you your healing.

Stage 2 of sit-with-it (requirements)

First, in order to *SIT-WITH-IT,* one must be READY—you must have a visceral (deep) desire to change. Second, you must have a BELIEF that change is possible, vital and needed. Third, you have to DECIDE change is needed. Fourth, you have to COMMIT to going through the *sit-with-*it process as outlined. Fifth, you must PLAN and STRATEGIZE—much like an army general.

In summary, to *sit-with-it* begins with a desire and belief, which is then fueled by a decision to make a commitment to a plan/strategy so that there is a permanent change in your lifestyle. You must understand that with change, comes growing pains as well as a passage through the uncomfortable. Your trust and hope in achieving your goals will come with practice.

Stage 3 of sit-with-it (tools)

For the remainder of this book, you will need a journal for making entries. Your journal will also serve as a reminder/refresher for when you finish reading this book. You will keep your journal in a place where you can see it at all times, because you will be making changes and adjustments on your way to weight loss and its maintenance. In fact, keep this book nearby as a reference if you hit the *relapse* stage, before it gets out of control.

Now, take out your journal, and make five lists. The first will list obstacles that could possibly derail your intentions (i.e., time restraints, family involvements or not truly being ready to make changes). Be honest. The second list will outline what it *costs* you to be overweight (i.e., loss of job opportunities, higher earnings, stamina, vitality, social engagements, health or sex). The third list will outline the *benefits* of being overweight (i.e., not much is required of you, you get to be lazy, you get off the hook for a lot of responsibilities, chores, etc.). The fourth list will outline the benefits that could be achieved with weight loss (i.e., being healthier, stronger, faster, improved quality of life, more social outings, etc.). The fifth list is outlined in stage 4 and suggests strategies that would take about 5-10 minutes of your time daily.

Look at your first four lists and see what you are willing to give up in order to gain and conversely, what you are willing to keep in order to gain. The truth may be scary, especially if you choose to remain overweight. But the important thing here is that you will now know what you did not know before about yourself and how you do what you do. From here, you can then choose to accept what you have found or choose not to accept what you found. Then, you make a decision for change or no-change. If you choose to do something about your numerous excuses, read on. If not, go ahead and put the book down for a later time when you are ready, *coachable* and believe that change is needed.

Stage 4 of sit-with-it (strategies)

This is a mindful stage. This is your opportunity to be creative and renewed. Open your mind and your journal, listing things you can do besides eating (because eating is a verb, an action word) and DO those things. If you "can not think of anything," ask others for suggestions. I recommend you come up with a list of *at least* ten things you can do when you recognize an emotional void or *hunger*. Personalize your list. Do not list things that you know are not possible financially or environmentally. Your new action list may look something like this: "When I am bored, horny, sad, disappointed, or happy, and it is not one of my pre-planned meal times, here are some things I am capable of lovingly doing: _____"

1. Take a walk (regardless of the weather; dress appropriately) by yourself, with a family member, friend, spouse, significant other or pet.
2. Build something, or take up a new hobby (sew, knit, crochet).
3. Work in your garden or start one.
4. Read a book.
5. Put a puzzle together.
6. Write in your journal.
7. Call a friend.
8. Write a letter or attend a meeting.
9. Do your homework.
10. Plan an event.
11. Do chores around the house (you, your family, or roommate will appreciate this);
12. Form a group or find an individual to whom you can be accountable—people who will be truthful with you. Family, with their good intentions may not want to hurt your feelings and therefore become enablers rather than truthful accountants.
13. Keep a food journal/diary, recording everything you put in your mouth, along with the date, time and serving size/amounts.
14. Read your food labels and choose appropriately.
15. Purchase and use a food scale for more accurate measurements (cooked weights of meats).
16. Weigh yourself weekly to avoid excessive weight gain without accountability and recognition.
17. Reward each stage of accomplishment with something other than food.
18. Deal with issues as they occur and refuse to use food as a comfort.
19. Schedule regular maintenance sessions with your counselor/therapist, registered dietitian, or physician, as appropriate.
20. Recognize when you are in denial.
21. Keep updated on healthy eating information/tips.
22. Continue some daily physical activity consistent with your licensed professional's (physician, physical therapist, personal trainer, etc.) recommended routine.
23. Be physically active daily or at least 6 days a week for 10-15 minutes (initially).

24. Keep vigil over your intake and make adjustments before you are out of control.
25. Consult your registered dietitian as frequently as necessary, in order to reassess caloric intake as each stage of weight loss is accomplished (e.g., -10 lbs, -20 lbs).
26. Encourage others with your success, examples and words.
27. Become an encourager to someone else.
28. Set the example for your family and friends.
29. Train for something (a 5K, 10K, marathon, relay).
30. Teach an aerobics or yoga class or work to become a personal trainer.
31. Commit to a life-time of good nutrition practices.
32. Bring a healthy dish to the cook-out, office party, picnic or pot luck.
33. Plan your meals and your days in advance. This way, when you smell or see that tempting food item, you can recall previously made plans.
34. Honor yourself, your body and your word.

The list is endless and you have to be its author because only you know where your interests lie. If it means purchasing a treadmill, elliptical or stationary bike, DO it.

Strategizing, before being placed in a tempting position, works. For instance, if I know I will be attending a party around dinner time, I am more mindful of what I consume at the breakfast and lunch meals so that I would not have gone *overboard* if I had a little extra at the dinner meal. If you have not planned your day, it is easier to fall prey to the stimuli around you. To help with this, I developed the affordable Tri-Part-U® wellness solution meal plan.

When you commit to your healthy living goals and the strategies you have devised to help you meet those goals, the rewards are great. Just do it. In order for any weight loss to be effective, you have to just do it. You have the power to choose to **be** your commitment, just as you have the power to choose to get out of bed everyday and go to work, because you believe you need to earn a living. Take control by choosing to live the healthiest you know right now. This involves a commitment to making nutritious food choices, improving your emotional health and increasing your level of physical activity.

Then, look for a return on your investment. The payoff can only pay in triple digit returns:

- Better sex life
- More energy
- Improved health
- Happiness
- Increased self-esteem
- Increased self-efficacy
- Decreased risk factors
- Healthier family
- Healthier outlooks
- More fun in your life
- More active retirement years
- Personal growth
- Physical/emotional/spiritual maturity
- Improved relationships
- More satisfaction with your life and choices
- More in control
- Stronger
- Inspired and inspiring

The list is long—write your own script and make it a winner! You choose. At this point, you should be at the *preparation stage* of change, with a strategy and a plan.

Chapter 5

The only way to have the life you dream is to be the life you dream

The development of Sit-with-it

The *how to* of the *sit-with-it* concept was birthed two years after attending a transforming seminar. The work done in the seminar radically transformed my life and indirectly the lives of my clients. The roots started to grow after I began to recognize the commonality of issues that plagued my clients, after so many years of teaching weight loss.

To understand the common thread, draw a tree and label each part. For example, each branch represents an automatic behavior (eating chocolate). You are the tree's roots ("I"). The tree's trunk is one of your core beliefs (I should eat when I'm stressed). Then, write a usual action you take in response to the *thought*, "I'm stressed." For example, when Janice wants something, she pulls together her thoughts from the roots. It begins with "*I am stressed.*" Then she rationalizes it with *I should* or *I deserve* (ex. "I should not be stressed."). She then pictures a comforting behavior like, "eating chocolate will make me feel better" (and eats it). As you see, it began with a recognition of what she was experiencing (ex. *stress*), followed with a rationalization/justification (I am stressed and I should not be). Followed with the verdict, "*I need chocolate because I am stressed*, which expresses itself with a practiced behavior (*eats chocolate*).

Part of what makes a tree strong is time and depth (how far down the roots go) and begin with you ("I"). The rationale behind the *shoulds*, wants, and desires are deeply rooted. They develop during your lifetime as a way to cope with your environment. For example, you cried and your caregiver gave you a bottle, you cried again and received another bottle or oral treat (e.g., cookie) to make you feel better. Eventually you made the association that to feel better you have to put something in your mouth. And since everyone around you is smiling after a meal, you draw the conclusion that food is the answer. Not just that, but doesn't everyone rave over Nana's freshly baked apple pie or mom's special corn bread? If you experience this enough times over the course of your childhood, your response to stress can cause your roots to get pretty embedded in food.

As adults, using food to decrease stress works because it is widely accepted. Isn't there some eating related celebration at least once a month, not to mention the fact that we need to eat daily? This is how it became such an easy and safe, but bad, habit to start. But, the opposite also is true. You may have come from a home where crying was more tolerated and alternate forms of soothing were utilized. So now, your stress response is rooted in other things (e.g., work, play, sleep or exercise).

You might be wondering: "How do I go about finding out the girth of my tree; or what does each ring represent; or, how did it get there?" I found help from authors such as John Bradshaw, PhD and Maxie C. Maultsby, Jr., M.D., a pioneer of Rational Behavior Therapy (RBT) and other therapeutic approaches.

For many of you, finding out why you do what you do may be sufficient to get you on track to healthy eating and weight loss. For others, you may find that the issue isn't "Do I have to lose weight?" But rather, "How do I handle the temptations that wash over me, when I am eating what I know I should not be eating or eating too much?"

The solution lies with *sitting-with-it* while you are in the mist of the temptation. As you stand in the midst of the madness, claim it. Call it what it is. For example, I like to joke that I am a "recovering chocoholic," because in the past, when I craved chocolate, chocolate was all I saw and dreamed about. When I was in a chocolate crave, I was giddy with knowing just how good it would taste. But, after going through the *sit-with-it* process, after purchasing it, and while transporting it in my car, I would ask myself, "How long do I have to walk on the treadmill for one serving?" Then, after I bargained with myself, I would eat it and get on the treadmill sometime before going to bed that day—just walking during a commercial break. Why? Because there was no guilt attached to having eaten it, once I knew I had balanced it with exercise. (Some may dispute this and call this an eating disorder, but isn't overeating disordered eating?). The thing to capture here, is that you want to be free to eat conscientiously without guilt (guilt is a common trigger to overeating). Eventually, when the desire for chocolate arose, I would ask myself, "Will I be able to find time to get on the treadmill tonight?" If the answer was, "No," I *freely* and *simply* gave up my thought about chocolate. Over time my cravings for chocolate stopped running me.

This example illustrates the thought processes you will automatically go through, but you have to be willing to keep your word. In this example, I knew I had to walk on the treadmill before the night was out. What are some tangible deals you can make with yourself that you know, and are willing to follow through with? And, are you committed to following through with your commitment to being healthy and following healthy practices? In this example, a 10-15 minute exercise was my *commitment* if I had already exceeded my daily caloric requirements. I don't obsess on calories because my mind is trained to eat healthier. Today, due to the distances I run, others find it hard to believe that I primarily walk one mile per day on my off-training days and my weight does not fluctuate from its norm during race season.

You may find that working with others in a group who you can call on during your tempting times, may be helpful. You may even find that a buddy club may help you, where you talk on the phone while engaged in an exercise (i.e., walking on a treadmill, or riding a stationary bike). You may even live close to someone who you can partner with to go for a walk, a bike ride, or run, at a certain time and frequency.

The most effective strategy is to remove excuses to your commitments to health. It doesn't matter that you have worked all day or have kids or spouse to care for. Manage your time in such a way that you create a space to meet your needs and that of your family's. Because when you are six feet under, the world still turns and the people and things you leave behind will still be there. So, drop the excuses, plan, strategize and *sit-with-it*.

For starters, post notes all over your home reminding you of your commitment. It can simply say, "*Sit-with-it.*" Post it on your refrigerator or pantry door, bathroom mirror, front door or work area. Why? Because there will be many times when you will forget what your goals are and this will serve as a reminder. Also, start to notice the times you read the signs and push them to the back of your mind, so that you conveniently *forget* what your commitment is.

Then, plan an event to celebrate each successful week you reach your goal of *sitting-with-it*. This way, it will remain fresh in your mind. If finances are a concern, join a weekly *sit-with-it* support group to keep you focused and generating new ideas.

Get into the habit of asking, "What are the benefits of being healthy?" And, conversely, "What is the cost to my health when I overeat?" My friend

Tom once said that, "Cravings are like stray cats, they leave when you stop feeding them."

From a psychological perspective, and according to Dr. Maultsby, "Say what you mean and mean what you say." He argues semantics and one begins to understand that semantics is everything. In his *Five Rules of Rational Thinking,* he expertly shows that the dialogue we have with ourselves is life-changing. His therapeutic work using RBT, among many things, is a comprehensive, quick-acting cognitive-behavioral approach that looks at our emotional ABC's. *A* is the activating event, *B* is the belief you have about *A,* and *C* is the feeling you have, or behavior you act out, because of your belief about *A.*

Further clarification came from going through the process outlined by John Bradshaw, therapist and author, in *Healing the Shame That Binds You* and *Home Coming: Reclaiming and Championing Your Inner Child.* I added to my understanding of the deeper layer of the emotional ABC's with my own inner child work, which quickly effected further beneficial changes in me. I saw the indirect benefits in my clients who were able to transform their own lives because I had created a space of being non-judgmental. Wives began to bring their spouses to me for nutritional counseling and I found that it became natural to pass on to them a natural inquisitiveness with regard to doing their own inner work. Then, friends started to refer their friends, and the benefits of the *sit-with-it* concept burgeoned and solidified itself as an effective weight loss tool, especially with my strong background in the field of foods and nutrition with an emphasis on weight loss counseling and as a registered dietitian. It took on a life of its own. It began to be my mantra for encouraging my clients. Once I gave it a name, its structure began to take shape. I found myself saying, "*SIT-WITH-IT*" and my clients knew what it meant. It had broken the counselor/client barrier. At times, tears were shed as defenses fell and awareness broke through. Clients were able to identify that their own belief systems were contributing to the sabotage of their weight loss goals. I found my clients to be encouraged, supported and motivated to reach their goals. For the first time since our initial consult, I heard strength, resolve and love in their voices. *Sit-with-it* works without pills, supplements and food-crutches.

In *Homecoming: Reclaiming and Championing Your Inner Child,* Bradshaw observed that, "It is the wounded inner child who forms the core belief system. By age-regressing into the inner child's trance, it is possible to change the core beliefs *directly and quickly.*" Also, "Once the core material is formed, it becomes the filter through which all new experiences must pass" (Bradshaw).

In the end, the clients that lost weight and maintained it had improved self-efficacy, energy and self-esteem (not to mention higher incomes from job promotions). Their resolve and commitment to making healthy lifestyle changes, and sticking to them, was proof that people can successfully lose weight and maintain it when they chose to *sit-with-it*. Yes, there were times when they got away from it, but they were able to reconnect when they reconnected with their designated support person/group. This is why if you do not have a support person, it is advisable to get into a support group that is committed to each other. You may also find it beneficial to work with a competent counselor/therapist who specializes in cognitive behavior therapy.

Now, stop and re-read the definition of *commitment* found in Chapter 1 because it appears that when people are at first experiencing weight loss, they appreciate the hand-holding, leading and encouragement. But for some, once they give up on themselves and the support person/group continues with the encouragement and support, they tend to back off, show resentment, and come up with excuses which by then, have already been identified as their "story." The thing to do, therefore, is to make a commitment that whoever is going to support you, you will accept the support and encouragement graciously regardless of how you are feeling; because of your initial commitment. If you fall into a rut or unhealthy familiar patterns, take the time to recognize and acknowledge that the old familiar pattern is causing you to be where you are. Go through the *sit-with-it* process to get back on track and away from relapse. If you can hold on to this concept, you will be better prepared to handle those "vulnerable" moments and get through.

When you decide to *sit-with-it*, all areas of your life will be affected. Like anything else, if you work it, it works. To sit on the stands and be a spectator will not get you the rewards you seek. Like all good athletes, you have to be in the game. Choose to be an active participant and *sit-with-it*.

Go beyond the "wall"

The *sit-with-it* concept is about getting beyond the wall of denial and resistance. For example, you will notice that when you are in the throes of an obsession, you are thinking about what you want to eat and how it tastes. You think about the many pieces you are going to cut it into as you go through all the reasons why you should have it or why you deserve it. You bargain with yourself that you will exercise more the next day. You even work out the details of how you are going to go to the store and purchase it—right down to how you are going to ask for and then pay for it (cash or credit). Stop! Fight the urge and get up and do something different.

Identify what you are feeling and acknowledge that the saboteur in you wants to prove that you can not do it. Recall that once you start to eat that food, you become aware that the first taste does not last. And that is what keeps you eating. You are trying to prolong the taste. The only thing that stops you is the uncomfortable feeling of being too full: it takes a negative reinforcement to stop you. The sad thing is that if you do not get a hold of this now, you will only continue to eat. Your stomach will continue to stretch to accommodate the new demand and before long, it will take greater and greater amounts for you to feel *full*.

Choose to stop the madness and masochism! Go to the nearest mirror and reaffirm yourself and the hard work you have done to this point. Picking up this book was probably your first step. *Sit-with-it!* Use the principles of RBT to confront the saboteur's litany. Take back control and do the healthy thing. Recognize that you are on a mission and that your mission is to be healthy. You will be uncomfortable at times, but do not succumb to the temptation of giving in. You know how badly you will feel the next day, or the next moment. Recall the feeling of being powerless and CHOOSE to be different and do differently. Become a health food and life fitness connoisseur. Remember, your taste buds can only register so much taste and then it becomes abuse and you have lost your first love—the enjoyment out of the first bite.

Tips

Before you can begin to *sit-with-it* you have to do some pre-planning. First, you have to recognize that when you say to yourself, "I am hungry," (especially after eating a complete meal), that is not a true physiological *hunger*. Instead, you may be hungry for companionship, love, warmth, affection, appreciation, recognition, or intimacy. You may be experiencing, among many things, any of the following: happiness, fear, rejection, loneliness, sexiness, relief, sadness, anger, anxiety, nervousness or boredom. Recognize that you have automatically trained yourself to convert these feelings into hunger feelings, and therefore you eat because it is safer to do so, than to experience what is. I can not enumerate the many times I have heard my clients say, "I eat for comfort." Yes, you may have an emotional hunger, but not a physiological hunger.

Recognize exactly what it is that you are feeling and the thoughts (*B*'s) that are supporting that feeling. Then, if you are lonely, *sit with* the feeling of being lonely. This means that for a moment, experience what the loneliness feels like. Enter it. Question its position and power. Assess it from all different angles with the goal of *not* making it *bad*, and then choose a non-food related activity to deal with it. For example, if you walked on your treadmill during TV commercials in a 2-hour program, you could possibly burn 50-60 calories (varies by intensities, or incline). That is a potential of 600-700 calories burned during one TV show. And remember, to lose weight daily, you have to spend more calories than you consume. Be careful however, that you do not fall into the trap of thinking that since you have exercised you need more food. No. The purpose of exercise is to promote weight loss and physical fitness by using the fat stores you already have for energy.

Therefore, acknowledge/validate the true hunger and you will see that it goes away with awareness and acceptance. If you did not acknowledge what you were feeling, you will find yourself unwittingly rummaging through the pantry in search of *feeding* the hunger feeling. You may even find yourself going through a number of different food items because what you ate "just did not hit the spot," so you kept searching through bags of cookies, cakes, candies, chips or an added food serving. However, when your stomach is stretched to its limit, you will find that your search temporarily ends. Temporarily, because what you resist persists. In another unguarded moment, the feeling returns to haunt you and you start to eat inappropriately again.

In summary, to *sit-with-it* requires: 1) recognition that your thoughts are behind your emotions and feelings of hunger; 2) your devising a list of alternatives to do rather than to eat; 3) planning your meals and physical activities daily; 4) committing to your plan; and 5) doing it—*sitting-with-it*.

Remember, when you *sit-with-it*, you are honoring yourself by demonstrating emotional good health, focus and self-love.

In order to have the thought processes that will facilitate the *sit-with-it* process, one first has to get emotionally healthy. If possible, meet with a trusted counselor or therapist. Otherwise, one of the quickest ways found to accomplish this is with Dr. Maultsby's RBT: emotional *ABC*'s. The following exercise is an example. It is designed to help you become aware of the self-talk that goes on in your head so that you can change the self-talk to produce the desired outcomes and keep you on track to meet your healthy goals. However, for RBT to work, you must truly want to make changes, or else, become anchored to what is known.

Chapter 6

Bread of deceit is sweet to a man; but afterward his mouth shall be filled with gravel.

(Proverb 20:17)

Stage 5 of sit-with-it (the mind process)

At my weight loss seminars, I teach going through the *sit-with-it* process, along with the Tri-Part-U® wellness solution approach to weight loss. At these workshops, I am usually asked, "Why can't I eat the *frivolous food* (refer to the *Tri-Part-U*® meal plan) everyday?" My response is, "When do you want to start seeing results?" Think about it. If you allow yourself to continue to eat the way you are eating now, how could you expect to see any changes or see change quickly? You will quickly come to find that when you make behavioral changes, your *cravings* change. Before you are able to *sit-with-it,* however, there are a number of steps to take. These basic steps form the foundation of helping you keep your goals and enable you to visualize what is possible. You will see how your actions are dictated by your emotional ABC's and the corresponding change in beliefs that have to occur in order for change to become permanent. Let us start with these three simple yet essential steps in rapidly eliminating emotional habits, put forth by Dr. Maultsby.

1. ***People must completely reject the beliefs and attitudes that support the undesirable habits.*** For example, after I have reviewed a specific meal plan with an individual, I may be asked, "Will I feel hungry?" I

usually counter with, "How long did it take you to fill your stomach to its current capacity?" You see, this is a ruse. This question attempts to hide the uncertainty and fear that one is feeling. We will call the client 'Joan.' During our consultation, Joan began to see the changes that she had to make and she was not interested in making those changes. Joan wanted to be given the short version to weight loss. She expected to be told that she could just take a pill and the weight would melt off. You see, usually, by the time clients come to a registered dietitian, they are really hoping for a single solution and not the meal planning work they receive. They are looking to feel better about their behavior without having to do any work. I have even heard some clients say that they will "shake and tremble" if they do not eat to feel full (despite the numerous times they have been so busy at work they skipped a meal and did not "shake and tremble"). But once they face the underlying anxiety related to not eating, they are able to make the necessary changes without trembling and shaking. (Again, this precludes those who have been diagnosed with a medical condition and who require more stringent monitoring.)

2. *Because nature abhors mental vacuums just as much as it abhors physical vacuums, people must replace their old beliefs and attitudes with new ideas that they are willing to make their new beliefs and attitudes.* This is where the rubber meets the road. What are you committed to changing? Take out your list of at least 10 things that you are committed to doing in place of eating again after a meal and remind yourself of the wonderful health benefits you will experience.

3. *People must practice acting out their new ideas until those ideas become their new beliefs and attitudes. Then, and only then, will people have created the semi-permanent, behavioral unit called a new behavioral habit.* Now do one of those things you said you would do without rationalizing it away. Do it as if you have always been doing it. As you do the planned activity you effectively re-train your mind to choose this as an alternative to eating in response to false hunger. To prepare you for those tempting times, spend 5-10 minute each day visualizing doing one of the healthy activities. Then, when inappropriate feelings of hunger occur, you will be able to automatically switch gears. [Note: *Clients are encouraged to recognize we are all actors on life's stage, so pick a part and play it to receive its health and fitness 'Oscar' award.*]

Personally, I got started after I saw an unflattering picture of myself taken by my sister at a zoo with the kids. I was home-schooling my oldest daughter and did not have the luxury of joining a gym. So I decided to start exercising in my living room. I would picture myself in a one-piece full-length dance leotard that my sister had given me and I would commit to being able to fit into it and look fabulous! I had been a nutritionist for eight years by then, and it finally dawned on me that I had to change my eating and exercise habits if I was going to make progress. I literally jogged in place for a half-hour each day, and then added various exercise videos to my routine. When I moved to Durham, North Carolina to start my dietetic internship, I looked for a community that had a fitness center and running/walking path. I created an environment where continuing my commitment to increased physical activity was always in my awareness, and I continued to set new physical fitness goals and challenges annually in order to improve my level of physical fitness. I trained for, and ran my first marathon at age 35. Now, when I travel, I purposefully look for accommodations that have a fitness center.

From both personal experience and the results obtained by my clients, I can say to you that once you go through the steps to replace old habits and form new, healthier ones, you will be on your way to losing the weight and keeping it off. Remember, you must think and act out your new beliefs consistently in order for it to become normal and natural (i.e., believe you are a fitness and nutrition buff—eat healthy and exercise daily). Dr. Maultsby warns, "Without enough time or practice, no new learning occurs."

Before reading further, pause, take out your journal and write down any arguments you may have to the above three outlined statements. Take your time and be as truthful with yourself as possible before going on.

Now, ask yourself the following questions to challenge any old beliefs that caused you to act out the old behavior of overeating. These questions are adapted from Dr. Maultsby's *Five Rules of Rational Behavior:*

1. Is your inability to lose weight based on obvious fact?
2. Does your current weight best help protect your life and health?
3. Does your current weight best help you achieve your short—and long-term goals?
4. Does your current weight best help you avoid your most undesirable conflicts with other people?
5. Does your current weight best help you feel the emotions you want to feel?

If you have looked deeply and have done the work in the previous chapters and truthfully answered, "Yes" to three or more of these questions, you can put down this book, as you do not see a need to make changes and may be at the *pre-contemplative stage* of change. If however, after doing the deep inner work required, you truthfully responded, "No" to three or more of these questions then read on and apply the next *ABC* exercise to your particular situation. (You could use the *ABC's* or arguments you came up with against the first three statements above).

Sit-With-It ABC exercise

For example, in the past, this occurred after Jill just ate a meal:

Activating event: Jill gets upsetting news.
Belief: I am stressed and I need a snack.
Consequence/feeling: She feels hungry and eats.

In this example, one would think that feeling upset is what made Jill hungry, but in reality it was her belief that she needed a snack that caused the *hungry* feeling. The *ABC* concept reveals that we behave based on what we believe and that certain events trigger those beliefs. For example, if you grew up in a family that used food for comfort, you will find yourself eating when you feel uncomfortable or stressed, even when you are not hungry, just by association.

Now after learning about her emotional *ABC's*, in the same situation, Jill becomes aware of what she is thinking and acts differently.

Activating event: Jill gets upsetting news.
Belief: I don't need a snack right now. I am upset and
                                        I will find another way to manage this stress.
Consequence/feeling: Jill calls a friend or goes for a walk.

Recognizing that your thinking is causing you to feel and behave the way you do, enables you to *sit with* your commitment by changing your thoughts and choosing alternatives. In this example, Jill identified what she was *thinking*. She recognized that her feeling of hunger was generated by her being upset and telling herself she needed a snack and should eat. She reshaped her thought to a more rational one that would help her meet her desired goals. She chose to ask herself the five rational questions and challenged her previously held belief. She followed up her new belief by reiterating her goals to herself and took the steps to help her meet her goals. In other words, she followed up with action.

The more rationally you do this exercise (by asking the five rational questions), the more quickly you will find that *you are more able to appropriately identify true physical hunger*. When you *sit-with-it* you effectively cut off any other obsessive thought you might have had about eating that comfort food. Robert Ellis, author of Rational Emotive Therapy (RET), maintains that people can best accomplish this goal by avoiding preoccupying themselves with *A* by acknowledging and yet resisting the temptation to dwell endlessly on emotional consequences at *C*. For example, "Oh, that would taste so good."

The goal is that by the time you have gone through the steps outlined above, and reminded yourself of your goals, you will no longer be around the temptation physically or psychologically.

Now, take out your journal and write down the *ABC's* of the particular situation(s) in which you find yourself overeating. There will be different activating events (*A's*), and it is therefore very important to be able to recognize them. In our workshop or while in a support group setting, you may be able to recognize other activating events you probably did not recognize as occurring because it was so habitual. Process each "*B*" with the five rational questions, and write out the *new* rational "B" and the new "*C*" (how you will feel with the new "*B*").

Using the above example ask yourself the following:	
Example 1	Example 2
1. Is eating a snack an obvious fact?	1. Is not eating a snack an obvious fact?
2. Does my eating a snack best help protect my life and health?	2. Does my not eating a snack best help protect my life and health?
3. Does eating a snack best help me achieve my short—and long-term goals?	3. Does not eating a snack best help me achieve my short—and long-term goals?
4. Does eating a snack best help me avoid my most undesirable conflicts with other people?	4. Does not eating a snack best help me avoid my most undesirable conflicts with other people?
5. Does eating a snack best help me feel the emotions I want to feel?	5. Does not eating a snack best help me feel the emotions I want to feel?
Did you answer "No" to 3 or more?	Did you answer "Yes" to 3 or more?

If you answered "No" to three or more questions in Example 1, then eating a snack is an *irrational* thought. If you answered "Yes" to three or more questions in Example 2, then to *not* eat a snack is a more *rational* thought.

It may seem too simple to be true, but going through this thought process works. The most difficult part of this exercise may be in *sitting-with* the feeling you are experiencing and validating it. Gestalt therapy is based on the premise that *awareness itself is therapeutic.* But I like to add, "When you are ready to do something with the awareness."

So, as you: 1) reject the beliefs and attitudes that support the undesirable habits; 2) replace your old beliefs and attitudes with new ideas; and 3) practice acting out your new ideas until they become your new beliefs and attitudes, you would have effectively created a new behavioral habit. This is the goal of the *sit-with-it* process—that when you are tempted to overeat or not exercise, go through the *ABC* steps and then *sit-with* the positive outcomes.

Chapter 7

Sticks and stones may break my bones, but names will never harm me.

The mind games we play with ourselves

"She is so fat!" "You are so big that . . ." The cruelties of childhood probably still haunt many of you. I am sure you could finish that sentence 100 times over. You could probably write a book on all the fat jokes you have heard in your lifetime, or you could list the derogatory names you have privately called yourself. You know firsthand that not just sticks and stones, but *words*, can also harm you.

The American College Dictionary defines fat as "having much flesh other than muscle; fleshy; plump" (1963). From this point forward, choose not to react negatively when someone calls you *fat*. *You* are not fat, but you are carrying a lot of extra weight in the form of body fat—adipose tissue. You know you call yourself *fat* when you look in the mirror. So, rule #1 is to choose to stop using name-calling as an eating trigger—excuse #1 of 1 million—you use negative self-talk so you can feel bad about yourself and justify food as your *comfort*.

How many excuses do you need to justify an extra cupcake or a candy bar, or whatever your "comfort" food is? Tired of lying? Here is the cycle:—hurt feelings → excuse to eat → eat → eat → feel bad about eating→ eat some more because of feeling so *bad* ("Might as well finish because, I have already started on this bag of chips"). In other words, the negative self-talk feeds the behavior, then throws you into a feeling of low self-worth, where you then look to food to comfort you. It is a vicious cycle that feeds itself. So if you are eating for comfort, it is time to start processing hurts and disappointments differently.

Weight loss research reveals that most people who gain weight and seek weight loss get depressed for a number of reasons. Again, there is no panacea or quick fix. Weight loss will take time. How long? Look at the time it took you to gain it, and it will depend on how much weight you have to lose. It requires commitment, change in core beliefs, motivation, accountability and responsibility. But most importantly, it requires facing the truth about the hard work ahead of you and making new commitments.

Do away with the excuses and myths, and replace them with commitment. Refuse to stay a prisoner, trapped in your own body, and seek release. It seems that slavery was eradicated from our civilized society but not in our bodies and minds. Free yourself from the slavery to food and immediate self-gratification. Resist the urge to fall prey to the enemy of overeating—sealing your coffin with heart disease, type-II diabetes, high blood pressure and cardiovascular disease—not to mention the inability to enjoy your life to its fullest potential.

Get off the circular treadmill to nowhere and *CHOOSE*. Choose to break out of your prison of "feeling bad" and enter a world of choice and power. You can do it today, right now, by committing yourself to following the principles outlined in this book. Take charge of your life! Choose a new attitude and wipe away life-long excuses from your memory board. Begin by telling yourself the truth. Give yourself a new *mantra* and allow the chorus from the song, *Voice of Truth*[1] by Casting Crowns, to be your new mantra:

> But the giant's calling out my name
> And he laughs at me
> Reminding me of all the times
> I've tried before and failed
> The giant keeps on telling me
> Time and time again. "Boy you'll never win!"
> "You'll never win!"
> Chorus:
> But the Voice of Truth tells me a different story
> The Voice of Truth says, "Do not be afraid!"
> And the Voice of Truth says, "This is for My glory"
> Out of all the voices calling out to me
> I will choose to listen and believe the Voice of Truth.

I am sure you have heard it said that what you resist will persist, and what you uncover diminishes in its power to control you. It is true. Face your tiger. Stop and take the time to uncover the truth about your underlying beliefs that contribute to your weight gain/excess. It is time to clean out your arsenal of excuses and storytelling, and replace them with new beliefs and loving affirmations.

Value yourself more than your addiction

When it comes to your health and wellness, you are the patient, the doctor and the pharmacist (adapted from financial analyst Suze Orman who said, when it comes to your "finances . . ."). She also said, "Replace the negative feelings about you being overweight, with a 'positive'/healthy attitude." Recognizing your triggers will help you take control of them. The clue to lifetime weight maintenance is in the process of seeking out your true self and your purpose for being here. Replace the negative body images with positive ones.

Why do we have to hurt for so long before we look for our healing? Either stop the madness, or step into it. Then you can begin to deal with the issues that caused it and thereby arrive at your healing. Life is precious—do not hasten your demise by treating your bodies so callously. Take the time to invest in maintaining yourselves—soul, mind and body—so you can do the best you can and reach your fullest potential. Stop the pain and cycle of sickness and disease. Honor yourself with a new commitment to good health, nutrition and exercise.

Chapter 8

The possible psychology of weight gain

Why do you eat beyond the point of satiety? Is it masochism or a band aid over an open wound? Is it avoidance or fear of who you want to be or acknowledgement of who you think you are? What is the negative internal dialogue that leads you to overeat? Is the pain you are experiencing so deep it overrides your body's *full* signal to the point of discomfort? When you refer to food as your comfort, are you trying to soothe a deep hurt that you have not given a name or voice? Is the wound of the inner child or toxic shame (described so well by John Bradshaw in *Healing the Shame That Binds*) within which re-affirms, "I can't; I am not worth taking care of myself, I am no good," or all those other inner voices that come up for you automatically?

One could also attempt to explain the psychology behind eating, using the operant and classical conditioning theory. For example, it could be when you first started eating (operant) you heard it was "good" with sounds of 'uhm' and possible comments from your important source figures (i.e., parent, guardian) who told you that what you were doing was a good thing. As you grew and were in social situations, especially from a source figure (Mom, Dad, grandparent) you again heard 'uhm' (reinforcement) and concluded to feel good (uhm—reinforcement) you had to eat or be eating. In operant conditioning, you learned to produce an operant (eating) behavior in response to a cue (uhm). So now, when you want to feel good, loved, worthy or accepted, you eat. This may sound very simplistic, but I believe, after the many years of teaching weight loss and listening to the common themes in my clients' stories, this is what is happening. Look how we reward our children with food to keep them quiet and engaged. Look at your family. When a child cries, the first thing reached for is the baby's bottle or pacifier—an oral fix. Recall the last time you were in a social setting with a crying baby. What did you do so others would not be annoyed with you or the baby? You fed it (or tried to feed it). The baby usually quiets down and now learns that when something is in its mouth, the caregiver is pleased and interprets this oral fix to mean all is well. Therefore, the behavior of having something in one's mouth is reinforcement to the feelings expressed by the infant/child and continues into adulthood.

For many, what was reinforced was *when I eat Mom, Dad, Nana, Grandma, or Grandpa are happy with me*; or *I am liked and accepted when I eat other people's food*. This can have a tremendous effect on a young child who does not feel good about himself.

As an adult, the individual continues to equate eating with being applauded or accepted by those important to them. Just look at the cook's face when you are asked to taste something the cook has made. You have effectively been *classically conditioned*. This is why as an adult, when others are telling you to lose weight, the overweight individual is saying on a subconscious level, "But that is the only way I feel good about myself, and the only way I will be liked." Even though on the outside, you know society is ostracizing you. You feel comforted in your behavior and see no real need to change: it is meeting one of your basic needs of acceptance. Through all this, you may have developed a core belief which says, "In order to be accepted, I have to be a people-pleaser" which plays itself out as you eat to satisfy the cook and yourself. Again, you incorrectly conclude food is your comfort despite the evidence to the contrary. Now in social gatherings with food, a previously neutral event becomes a conditioned stimulus and you behave automatically by eating without regard to the amount or consequence. Rational Behavior Therapy (RBT) helps you argue against this ingrained belief and helps you change your relationship with food by changing the core belief—but you must first identify the core belief. Then, the new belief changes the conversations you have with yourself and ultimately the behaviors.

On the other hand, maybe for you being overweight is like thumbing your nose at the next guy and saying, "See, look at me. I can do what I want.

I am in control. I am the big boss now." This may be because in your past, you felt your life was out of control. This belief could represent the fear that says, "Life is scary and uncertain." In response, you live as if this is your last day on earth because you really do not believe you will or should see tomorrow. You may even not want to see tomorrow. If this is the case, there may be some underlying depression that has not been addressed and would be best evaluated by a therapist, counselor, psychiatrist or psychologist. For others, in your past, you may have felt others controlled your life and in response to what you believe about the control others had on your life, you live recklessly without regard to negative consequences.

Attempt to answer these and many similar questions by *being* your word (refer back to Chapter 1: *Commitments re-defined*). When we are not keeping our word there is dissonance and the feeling of shame is experienced. We feel guilty for what we have consumed and to soothe our discomfort, we eat. We eat because we were uncomfortable, and to be uncomfortable is intolerable. The familiar is chosen. Herein lies the dissonance, because at this stage it is important for you to be able to go beyond the uncomfortable, and to *sit-with-it*. For some, you will be *sitting with* your commitment to identify what triggers your overeating. For another, you will be *sitting with* the commitment to simply listen to yourself—your instincts. And for someone else, you may be *sitting with* your commitment to exercise. Choose what you want to *sit with* and then *sit-with-it*.

Viewed another way, by making unhealthy choices, we choose to shorten our lives and make it more challenging than it needs to be. What will it take to make you see YOU are in the driver's seat of your life? We are on a journey called life and your eating and exercise habits (or lack of them) determine which roads are available to you. You desire happiness and contentment, but instead you take the road to depression and despair. You desire long life and health, but you steer towards disability and disease. You desire to wear a size 12, but choose a size 26. You desire to be skinny, but overeat and not exercise. You desire to be athletic and quick, but you choose to be out of shape and sluggish.

I want to encourage you to see life as a joy ride—a game. You design your own amusement park. You choose which ride you will enjoy each day. The choices are yours to make. No one and nothing can take that responsibility from you. Studies have shown a high connection between a past history of abuse and overeating. They suggest some may turn to food as a comfort and to build a wall of protection around themselves. And although this is obviously not the case in all instances, an argument may be made for the individual who may have been similarly traumatized, but who dealt with the trauma by becoming skilled in the marshal arts or kickboxing to protect himself/herself. They have both built a wall of defense but one is made of excess adipose tissue, versus muscle and agility. These individuals chose their defense, so let us not just stop at choice. Take it one step further to healthy choices. (Note: if you are a victim of abuse or trauma, please seek help—you are worth it.)

The possible anatomy of weight loss

Deprivation versus starvation: Could it be what throws us off behaviorally, is that we listen to the inner child voice that says "I want, I want?" For example, as a child we had no control over obtaining what we wanted. So now, as an adult, we say "yes" to the child within us. This makes it more difficult to tell ourselves, "It is okay to want something and it is equally okay to not always get what you want" because the feelings experienced as a child are fresh each time you *want* something. Start to identify other areas in your life where you are giving yourself what you want, to diffuse the overall impression you may NEVER get what you want. If not, when a *want* or *desire* occurs, you will see it through a filter of, *it is a need,* and a cascade of beliefs and emotions that require "comforting" will be generated.

To understand what is happening, stop and consider one of the steps to weight loss and its maintenance is healing the wounded inner child. Considerably, one of the possible struggles with weight loss is once the weight has been lost, the reason it is so easy to gain it back is stress hits and the coping habit of eating is triggered. The possible underlying stream of thought could be "we want something and we question our ability to get it." Therefore not to get it would be to deprive our inner child.

These same thought processes can lead to us overindulging our own children. If you are a parent, you know the struggles you face when your child(ren) asks something of you that you know you cannot afford or provide. In the same regard, denying yourself the extra serving or calorie-rich item you want is the same as telling your child, "no." The problem with saying, "No," is we feel inadequate because we are not able to meet our child's need. And here is where it gets blurred, because it is not that we are not meeting our child's **need**, but not meeting our child's **want**. In other words, our inability to meet that want may be financial. Then we move into "guilt mode" and make the want a "need" and give in.

Part of *sitting-with-it,* is identifying that part of the anatomy of weight loss is really a visceral response to protect your wounded inner child.

Why dieting does not work

When someone embarks on losing weight for the temporary purpose of fitting into a wedding gown, looking good for a class reunion or special vacation, or catching a potential mate, they are doomed to weight maintenance failure. The reasons are numerous but still, temporary. Inevitably, after the event or the relationship has started, the weight comes back on. In terms of relationships, we make our mate "wrong," for not "accepting us as we are," as we regain the lost weight we used to trap him or her with in the first place. What changed? What happened? The goal was short-term. You had no intention of continuing the *diet*. The thought never occurred to you that as soon as you returned to your old eating habits that caused the weight gain, the weight would return. You saw weight loss as magical: once the weight came off it would stay off on its own.

There is no getting around it: the truth is losing weight is not only hard work, it is continuous work. For example, Lance Armstrong did not win the Tour de France multiple times by only training once.

A frequent excuse I hear is, "I do not have will power." Well, I do not agree. You do have will power—but unfortunately, it is tied to a self-defeating core belief. If you believe you can not lose weight, your behaviors will lead to weight gain. For example, I have patients who come in with chest pains and who tell me it is not related to their excessive weight! They believe they do not have control over their health. They believe their health is passive and the illness just happened to them. So what are the chances of this individual losing weight? No chance. Would you work hard for something you did not believe in? Even now, if you are saying, "Well I m not that big," and your BMI is >25, according to the National Institutes of Health, you are at an increased risk for getting type II diabetes mellitus, hypertension and/or cardiovascular disease (to name a few). How do you want to spend your golden years? Strapped to a machine breathing for you, or, strapped in a seat belt as you enjoy multiple vacations and outings—both of which you earned equally with time? Choose to spend your time wisely.

The bottom line is, because *dieting* is temporary, most people quickly regain the lost weight and more. Further studies, leading to the NIH Clinical Guidelines on the Identification, Evaluation, and Treatment of Overweight and Obesity in Adults (1998) suggests, "most dieters regain their lost weight within 5 years of completing treatment." Currently, the general guidelines for weight loss are losses of 5-15 percent of initial body weight. Therefore, a weight loss goal of 5-10 percent your current weight over the next three to six months, with maintenance, is not unrealistic—since even a small weight loss is beneficial.

Weight loss is not solely about will power, but rather a belief in the fact that what you choose to eat and the physical activity you choose not to engage in, is not costing you your health, vitality, and current quality of life. In other words, you do not believe you are causing your own sickness and disease. Thus, weight loss is temporary because you really do not believe you "are what you eat." How you treat your body now WILL catch up with you. It is just a matter of when.

Remove your denial-colored spectacles, and take charge of your life. Therefore, the first stage of weight loss is to BELIEVE losing weight and maintaining its loss is really beneficial and necessary. In fact, your life depends on it.

Chapter 9

Will Power: If I have the will, I have the power.

You might be saying to yourself it requires will power, dedication, and discipline to lose and maintain your weight. However, I say you already have that will, power and determination. The core foundation of your "willpower" and/or discipline and/or determination, is your belief. You believe you are entitled to or deserve more. And not wanting to deprive yourself (you have earned it)—you eat. You also believe if you do not eat, you will starve (even though you are carrying around extra weight). This has been proven with individuals who in the past have said, "Oh, if I do not eat, I will starve or pass out." These same individuals will get the bariatric surgery, in some cases having gone from a 3,000-4,000 calorie/day diet to a 500-800 calorie/day diet, and guess what? They did not starve, or pass out.

I am convinced that whatever you *believe* will be the foundation of your will power and/or discipline and/or determination. For example, if I truly *believe* I will starve, then it would only be rational to eat, because no one wants to starve? Also if I believe I am depriving myself by not eating something, then I will act in accordance with that belief and eat something. Also, if I *believe* being healthy makes me feel and look good, I will choose foods and activities that promote that belief. Our beliefs control our behaviors (refer to Chapter 6). Therefore, we do those things we believe. It is like getting out of bed each morning to go to work—we believe it is necessary—to earn a living. Therefore, why not change your beliefs? From experience, cognitive behavioral approaches help clients to quickly change old beliefs so the new beliefs line up with the expected results—the dream. It makes no sense to dream up something we believe we cannot have. The dream materializes when you dream of something you believe you can achieve and you put into place the necessary processes to realize the dream. Ask any manager, CEO, leader or coach. That individual or team of individuals, have a dream they believe can be realized and the next step is to implement the necessary steps to make the dream happen.

This is no different. The next step is to create a belief system where you can achieve your dreams and your desires. The *sit-with-it* process is designed to help you meet those goals. When you *sit-with-it* you really face your tiger. Look at what you want and what you have to do to achieve it. Then, put into place those things to have it happen. For example, I hear clients say, "I want to lose weight." However, the missing piece is they do not believe they can lose weight and because they do not believe they can lose weight, they do not even have the capacity to rationalize some of the steps they can take to have the dream realized. I also hear, "I can't," "I do not have the will power," "I do not have the discipline," "You do not understand," "I am not like you," or, "I have been this way forever." The excuses go on and on. We have all heard them before, and we have all said them in one way or another.

Rewrite your old script. Read on to find out how. The benefits will exceed your weight loss goals and you will see other areas of your life open up. For example, debt-free living, being kind, charitable or being less reactionary. After you have outlined the strategies of how to accomplish one of your commitments when temptations arise, you apply the same steps to help you meet your goals. A lot of the success stories of my weight-loss clients have not just centered around their weight loss but on their experience of having greater emotional depth with their significant other, job promotions, career changes, and personal and financial fulfillment. The list is endless. The commitment we spoke of previously is the commitment to do the necessary work so you can *sit-with-it*. Once you *sit-with-it*, it becomes a part of your lifestyle. The fear of regaining the lost weight will no longer be valid because you would have successfully implemented the necessary steps to get you where you are and to keep you there. The *sit-with-it* concept embodies not just the physical, but the psychological and spiritual you. We are three parts—mind, body and soul. Each one depends on the others to be healthy. Therefore, it *only* makes sense to build up and keep all three areas healthy. You can, if you apply the principles set forth in this book. *Sit-with-it* and successfully achieve your short—and long-term weight loss and/or weight maintenance goals.

Chapter 10

Reward each success with positive affirmation

What is there to ponder? The bottom line

The bottom line is whatever you choose to do regarding lifestyle changes, make sure it is something you can do for the rest of your life in order to ensure weight maintenance.

Remember, weight loss and its maintenance is about personal responsibility. It relies on your keeping your word (your promise) to yourself and your loved ones to care enough to do the best you can for yourself. To accomplish this, you must set realistic goals, work with a registered dietitian, therapist or counselor, personal trainer and your physician. As a team, they will help you get on track and support your efforts/successes.

Start out with one to two goals and advance appropriately. Each success should be followed with one to two more goals set. Successes should not be rewarded with food. Instead, buy a new outfit, jewelry, spend a day at the beauty spa, or plan a trip. For me, I rewarded myself with jewelry after I ran my first ultra marathon! In fact, as a "recovering chocoholic," I started running, so I could eat as much chocolate as I wanted, without wearing it on me! But now, I have reached the point I am so happy with my body for its excellent performance, all I want to do is give it good nutrition versus *consistent* "junk" food! It was, and now is, my way of saying, "Thank you," to my body for staying in good health, so I can work and earn a living doing what I truly love, engage in physical activities I really enjoy, and spend quality time with those dear to me. And now, I am residing in a body I consider beautiful and my ideal—my dream body.

The benefits of being healthy are exponential! I am a role model for my children and I am able to be their support and encouragement. My family's resources are not taxed (emotionally, physically, spiritually and financially). I am able to teach by example and word. They can deposit it in their storehouse of safety and trust. I am also more able to empathize with my clients and offer hope and encouragement. Best of all, I am able to maintain and boost my energy when it is running low or drops to empty. In sum, I treat this vessel God has given me the best I know how. I liken it to the man with the talents in the Bible (Matthew 25: 14-30) and the investment God (or your Higher Power) has given me, I have managed to the best of my ability, to maximize its return. This responsibility resides with no one else but me.

Another truth behind weight loss is you really have to believe the reason for what you are doing and have a health-oriented goal (and not just because you are going to a wedding or family reunion). Know the benefits your wellness goals will produce and look forward to the anticipated changes. If you are only trying to fit into a dress or suit for an occasion, once the event passes and there is nothing else to look forward to, the weight will return. Therefore, set both short—and long-term goals before the initial goal has been achieved. It is very important to know and believe being healthy is not only important, but possible. It will improve your overall health and quality of life.

Chapter 11

I have lived on an island with bridges, and I've never crossed them.
(Kate and Leopold)

How many of us can relate to the experience of wanting to lose weight but not doing what it actually takes to cross that bridge and have it happen? We may have tried temporarily, but have not gone the actual distance. We have not stuck to our goals with the diligence and fortitude of an athlete. We have all heard exercise is key in the weight loss and maintenance game, but we are still waiting for a magic pill or patch to be invented so we can ignore the hard work it really takes. It is my hope you will finally see you have the opportunity to cross bridges and get to the other side to a healthier you.

With the aid of your support person or group, therapist or counselor, begin to explore the psychodynamics of your past, present and future that allow you to continue to gain excess weight—and move on. Read self-help books, attend health-related seminars or workshops to further explore the issues that may surface for you. Look at the self-talk you engage in as you obsess on food. Look for the traps, triggers and excuses you use to give yourself permission to overeat. Recognize you are playing a deadly game because of the health complications, and the decreased quality of life to which you have allowed yourself to slip into. Notice how I said *slip*, versus *fall*, because to *fall* implies something occurred suddenly, when we all know gaining weight is a process.

We are all aware of the negative body image we see projected back to us when we look in the mirror. We alone know the diatribe of self-loathing and disgust we engage with ourselves, while on the surface pretending to be in control. We pretend no one will notice our excess weight and waste energy being angry with how society sees us. We even catch ourselves laughing at our own weight in the company of others, and may even tell a few "fat" jokes of our own as if to imply we are comfortable with our weight. We have so bathed ourselves in denial, we even believe the lies we have told others (e.g., it is hormonal, it is genetic, I am big boned, I just love to eat or, I just love food). Do not turn your anger inward—it leads to stress and weight gain. Instead, turn toward awareness, acceptance and healing.

I once heard it said, 'Trouble, like babies, grows larger with nursing." This is no different with regard to weight gain.

Chapter 12

Counsel in the heart of man is like deep water;
but a man of understanding shall draw it out.

(Proverb 20:15)

To begin

1. BELIEVE you can make a difference in your overall health. Look at changing how you eat and how you can increase your physical activity level. Make a realistic assessment of your current weight and what has contributed to its increase (resist the excuse, "My spouse is a good cook."). Look at the different ways you can incorporate moderate to intense physical activity into your daily lives (discuss with your physician as needed).
2. PLAN on a change of lifestyle. You can get caught up in the idea of losing weight without actually doing anything. You philosophize, strategize, and analyze; but remain in a rut. You will find, however, as soon as you have moved from the *preparation stage* to the *action stage*, you will pick up energy and the process gets smoother.

However, this is your most vulnerable time. You can be derailed at this point by well-intentioned loved ones, who may also be overweight. You may hear comments like, "You are getting too thin;" or "Do not lose any more weight—we will not be able to see you." Consequently, you may be left struggling with feelings of being deprived. You may begin to ruminate on thoughts like, "How come he can eat that and I can not? And before you know it, you have gone off track and given up your goal of being healthy and fit. This is why it is highly recommended you be involved with a loving and supportive weight loss group before starting your healthy living journey.

It is sad but true that even your staunchest supporter can be the very person who causes you to stumble. How? Why? Just look at what you had to do to get where you are. There were issues to be dealt with. You had to face your tiger and stand up to your fears. You had to make commitments to yourself and follow through. You had to alter your life so a creative and supportive environment could be established. Now you are probably questioning whether it was worth it. You may even have started dating and convinced yourself your mate should love you no matter what.

Your mind is going through endless rationalizations as to why you do not need to avoid "one more serving." Caution, as soon as these rationalizations occur, sound the alarm in your head. You are going through a vulnerable time, so tune into what you are feeling or experiencing and then *sit-with-it*. Do not be derailed. Review your healthy living goals and the steps you have taken to get you where you are. Write new goals if necessary and a plan of action to attain them. Stop in at your local support group or call your support person more frequently to get you through times of crises. If you do not have a local support group or person, consider starting or finding one.

Form a new relationship with food

Re-form a healthy relationship with food. Begin to see food as *fuel* versus *comfort*. Have you noticed you can not over-fill your car's gas tank? So why would you do it with the vehicle which makes it possible for you to afford the car? I am almost sure you do not want to rely on pills for the rest of your life. You would prefer to learn behavior change strategies to employ, to ensure that you can eat sensibly and satisfyingly in any situation. This is something you can take with you no matter where you go. You do not have to keep buying it, or replenishing it: it is free and yours forever. Wouldn't you rather spend your hard-earned money elsewhere than on hospital bills, medicines or supplements? I once stood in line with a woman who explained to me she needed the pills she was buying to help her keep the weight off—"Without them, I keep overeating." Personally, I would rather save my money for more enjoyable pursuits.

Look out for familial pitfalls

Unfortunately, some families have not always been very supportive, not because they did not want to be, but because they did not know how to be. Consequently, the weight loss goals were derailed. At times it may seem like our human tendency is to hold on to what we want or believe, rather than to get on board with another's plans." This can be seen as a form of "resistance." Even Jesus said, "A prophet is not welcomed in his own house." Your family is not trying to be mean, but think about it. When you know someone is good at something you are not, do you at first encourage and support them, or do you point out the many things they are doing wrong? Yes, you "nit pick." For whatever reason you do not try to build the person up, but rather you try to take them down with the rationalization you are helping them to remain "humble." It is as if helping them will force you to see the many changes you could have made for yourself but did not. How many times has a friend told you he was on a diet and you offered him a dessert or an extra serving? It will be no different with your family. This is why you have to be committed to your goals and their outcome. The support and encouragement you crave may or may not be found from your loved one, whom you feel should be your closest ally. Remember, just as you have issues, so do others.

The *sit-with-it* concept was borne out of this reality. There will be times when to *sit-with-it* is challenging and overwhelming not because you do not feel like doing the best thing for yourself, but because you see your significant other doing the opposite of what you are committed to doing. You may experience a variety of negative feelings (regret, resentment, anger, guilt, grief or shame). And, if you usually eat for comfort, this can easily trigger a relapse into feeding the *hunger*—the perceived negative feeling of deprivation, or lack of acceptance, or whatever it is you are experiencing. This is a very vulnerable time and emotional issues may cloud your judgment. This is where the expertise of a therapist or counselor may be beneficial in helping you keep your focus.

For example, you may go through some very sad moments as you grieve the loss of support from friends or family. In these times, you will find your outside support—group or person helpful. The temptation may come for you to begin to resent your loved one, friend or significant other, but do not go there! Look at your emotional ABC's (refer to Chapter 6), and replace the belief, "they are out to get you" or "they do not love me," with, "I am committed to the outcome of healthy living, and I choose to continue to honor myself with . . . ." Do not turn your anger and disappointment inward or toward your family. Use the energy and new-found resolve to continue to move you forward.

Sure, it would be nice to have a partner who shares the same goal(s); someone who will be there for you as you go through difficult times. But this is not always the case. Again, it would be nice, but it is not always possible. *Sit-with* this feeling. You can also choose to look at the humorous side of it as Bob Schwartz did. Schwartz is a running enthusiast and humorist. In *I Run, Therefore I Am NUTS!*, he writes, "I viewed one of my parental duties as a kind of Svengali nutritionist and appointed myself Chief Deputy of Diet. I figured I'd mold their eating habits and we'd soon be scarfing down chunks of wheat gluten and sucking on ginger cubes . . . Welcome to the real world of a kid's penchant for strawberry-flavored milk and glow-in-the-dark macaroni and cheese."

To *sit-with-it* means you recognize who YOU are and what YOU are about. What are YOU committed to? In time, the role model you become for your children, family and friends will ultimately pay off. Importantly, don't make them *wrong* and you *right*. Personally, I was thrilled when my eight-year-old daughter said, "Mommy, I get it now. I am not going to quit, I am going to keep on trying," after I had just finished running my first 100 mile race! At first, this concept might seem vain because of how we were raised, but when has it ever been vain to take care of ourselves? How could we possibly take care of others, if we let ourselves go? Even now, you may be able to take care of others, but for how long? How can you gift away your soul? Only you know the thoughts running through your mind. Only you know the act you put on, the play you orchestrate, or the true solace you seek.

Recently, as we were hanging out at home together at 8 o'clock in the evening, my 13-year-old daughter (who previously could not see the benefit of running), asked if she and I could go for a run together! I jumped up and put on my running shoes, grateful I had not dropped the ball on my goals to be physically fit.

Whatever you do, do not take on the sadness that will engulf you at times because you are like a *one-man show*. Just know you have embarked on a journey that may have a big send off, but may not end with cheers at the finish line. It is okay, s*it-with-it.*

Chapter 13

"Breaking old habits and forming new ones is sometimes a painful process. It is a change that requires the willingness to subordinate what you think you want now for what you want later. But this is the process that produces happiness."

(Covey)

Changing conversations with ourselves

Initially, you may have had conversations which sounded like this: "*I sure could use a caramel latte right now. It will be okay. I will substitute it for my soup at lunch later. I have the rest of the day to make it up. In fact, I will have less at my next meal.*" Before you know it, you have compromised your commitment to eating healthy and given yourself an excuse to eat what you wanted. Yes, you may be within your caloric goal, but missed your healthy eating goals. What is the big deal? If you do this enough times, you will find yourself so far from your goals you may end up giving up. At this point, the weight increases and in most instances, you may have gained more than you initially lost.

To *sit-with-it* means you go through the process outlined in Chapter 6 and remind yourself of your commitment to a healthier way of living and eating. You picture the end, the finish line. You ask yourself if giving in to eating that food or not exercising will help you reach your goals. Then do it—exhibit behaviors in line with your goals (e.g., you go for a walk instead of driving to the store). Do not try to talk yourself out of your decision, just do it.

For example, you want a piece of chocolate cake and it will be your second slice of the day. Stop and ask yourself the five rational questions and then ask yourself, "Why do I want another piece, after just finishing the first piece? Am I bored, lonely, or sad?" [Feelings will vary by situations]. *Sit-with* the idea, "I am bored." Now look through your journal of things to do when you are bored and choose to do one of them, rather than to eat the chocolate cake (refer back to Chapter 4). In time, in the act of doing something else, the desire to eat when you're bored disappears, because the boredom is now replaced with action. And with a sense of action, you are now in a position of control. You have provided your brain with information it can access the next time the situation comes up. Basically, without action your brain has no memory base to recall from.

[Caveat: Be aware if you return to the kitchen, you might be faced with the desire to eat again, and therefore it is important to have strategies. This is why it is not a good idea to put off washing the dishes until later—because you will have to return to the kitchen and another eating trigger may be set off!]

In the beginning, with individual—or group support, it is recommended you take the time to attempt to identify the underlying thoughts surrounding the negative feelings towards boredom (or whatever feeling you were able to identify that triggered the "hungry" feeling). I say negative, because it is usually something we perceive as negative or bad for which we seek comfort. When you are able to identify the underlying beliefs, you will be in a position of control and will be better able to diffuse the desire to eat.

Therefore, when I *sit-with-it*, I have a rational and objective conversation with myself. For example, at 5 a.m. in the morning when the alarm goes off, I can either say to myself, "It is too early, I will exercise later," and roll over and go back to sleep, or "You always feel much better about yourself after a workout and you only have to walk one mile. Besides, you will not get much more sleep anyway." With this thought I get out of bed, dress and go to the gym or get on my treadmill. And as promised, I feel much better about myself. Therefore, this is the conversation I choose to have with myself at 5 a.m. in the morning, because with this conversation, I reach my goal. You can do the same. But remember, if no action follows your new thoughts, good habits will not form.

Again, changing your self-talk to have the second conversation mentioned above is a process; but with practice, it becomes routine. Personally, when others find out about the distance races I run (marathons, ultra marathons, and ultra ultras), they usually ask me, "How do you do it?" And, my response has not changed—"I do not know how *not* to do it"—it has become routine. It is a healthy habit.

A particular client comes to mind when I think about exercise. Before Ben lost more than 100 lbs, he balked at my suggestion he attempt to walk one mile in 30 minutes. Now, he run/walks two miles per day, every day! I think the benefit of exercise is not just in the doing of it, but in the fact you took the time to do something good for yourself. The resulting psychological satisfaction far exceeds, in my opinion, the physical benefit of having done the exercise. I call this the psycho-social mind-body connection.

More examples of possible conversations

"I am going to do whatever I want, regardless of the consequences. I will deal with them when it happens." Obviously, if this is how you are thinking, the feeling generated is, resignation and the thought process to support it is, "To heck with it." Consequently, the behavior that will occur is for you to do what you feel like doing in the moment. *Sit-with-it* says that once you are aware of what you are thinking you pause, rethink your goals, go through your list of alternatives, and do one of them.

Capture that your temper tantrum is costing you your health and vitality and is robbing you of your rich existence. Conversely, a healthier conversation to have would be, "It would be nice to have a *banana split* (example), however I choose to only have half, or one-fourth, or none of it, because I am committed to my overall health and wellness." Having this conversation, your feeling is going to be one of accountability and control; your behaviors will reflect the belief, "Yes, I am responsible for my actions." The outcome/consequence is you act in moderation.

You might be saying to yourself, "When am I going to have the chance to just go home, sit down, relax and eat whatever I want? I have worked all day!" This can only be answered by the person who has arrived or does not have an issue in the evening time. For many, their most tempting time is in the evening after work. They just want to sit around and eat, do nothing and think about nothing. If this describes you, start to look around your house and make a list of everything that needs to be done in your home. If you have been meaning to wallpaper, scrap book, sew, redecorate, repaint, fix, repair, clean out the basement or garage, separate or take out winter, spring or summer clothes, then take out your journal and put it on your project list. Give yourself 15-30 minutes each evening to work on a project. If cost is an issue, look in sales papers for parts or get a home improvement book and learn to do a lot of things yourself; or partner with others who know how to do what you are trying to accomplish. For example, when I was working on my scrap book, I called my girlfriend and she loaned me a lot of the starting supplies. When I was hanging wallpaper, I called another friend and she showed me how. Then, I started hanging around the home improvement stores and looking at classes they offered as well as pricing parts and equipment for purchase and rental. So initially, what your evenings are going to look like is someone in the *preparation stage* of change. The energy you will generate just from the flow of ideas and planning will be enough to move you into the *action stage*. As you go through the processes, one step at a time, and complete projects, your sense of accomplishment will be unbeatable. Work on one project at a time. There is no rush: this is your therapy. Take your time enjoying these projects. Realize these actions will be the distraction you need to keep you away from food. Remember, you may be tempted to say, "I do not want to spend my evenings like this." But again, remember you are now committed to doing things differently than you did in the past.

In the past, you would probably have just sat around, eating and watching TV. You would have been bored into telling yourself, "I deserve this." The thing to identify here is because you were "working" earlier in the day, you felt the need to come home and do nothing versus something (note: even eating is something). The intended reward is your house will be in order and you would have experienced weight loss while developing healthier coping strategies. With practice and time, following the *sit-with-it* process will enable you to come home and just plop down, relax and take it easy with new, healthier behaviors. However, for right now, during this very vulnerable time, your options are going to look a little different.

The time will come when you look around your newly improved sanctuary—your house, your home—and appreciate its beauty because of all the things you have done to it and all the time you have spent on it. You do not have to be a homeowner to realize these benefits. Improvements can be made to borrowed, shared or rented spaces as well. By that time, you would have gone through the *sit-with-it* process and your old habit of sitting around eating will be only a memory. You would effectively have replaced the old memory of being a "couch potato" with being an active participant in your life and creating for yourself, an environment that is warm, inviting and fulfilling. And, YOU did it.

Also, it is important to note that you have to honor the gentle guidance you receive from your support—person or group with whom you have shared the goals to *sit-with*.

Further, resist the temptation to ask the "why" question? Because when you ask, "Why?" it prevents you from entering the space of rationally stopping and trying to identify what your core beliefs are. The "why" question just puts up a front and further spirals you into self-recriminations, guilt, and shame. This is not the intent of the *sit-with-it* process.

Chapter 14

The experience of sitting with it

You will recognize that as you *sit-with-it*, you will find yourself obsessing on the things you were committed to avoiding, like eating. You may find yourself strategizing on how to get what you want and then rationalizing why you should have it. Be aware this thought process will return you to your eating addiction. These thoughts and behaviors are usually followed by self-recriminations and promises to "do better" the next time.

To truly *sit-with-it*, once you recognize you are headed toward your addiction, you stop obsessing by choosing to do something different (refer to your list). You will naturally want to get what you want and purposefully not "*sit-with-it.*" So the challenge is to *sit-with-it*, get up, and write in your journal the feeling(s) you are experiencing. Become aware of what you need in the moment (for example, you may want to experience intimacy without sex—to just be held and comforted, or to be made love to slowly, or to talk heart-to-heart with someone you really care about, or to experience something which has been stuffed down for a long time). Become aware of the particular need that is trying to get lost in food and figure out another way to get it met. Some actions you could take include: writing a letter or a poem, reading a book, or calling a friend. If you are in a trusting relationship, share what you are feeling. If you do not feel comfortable doing so, suggest couple's—or individual counseling to your partner Whatever you do, *sit-with-it* and it will pass, not because you ignored it but because you acknowledged it and were proactive in dealing with it.

Tell yourself you are a winner on this new health journey and remember it is a process that takes time, commitment, practice, repetition AND action. Choose to be healthy and know and believe in your commitments. If you are asking, "Why can't I just do the basics to get by?" The answer is: the basics are not enough.

Remember, there are many possibilities to the anatomy of weight loss, including the possibility that the *full* feeling we experience after eating a very satisfying meal is symbolic of the lack of completeness we feel in our own lives: the lack of fullness we so desperately yearn for. So, as our stomachs stretch to the point of satiety and *uncomfortableness*, we get a strange satisfaction. To put one more bite in our mouth would be balancing between total lack of control and masochism—self-punishment. Then, as the feeling of lethargy creeps over us, we begin to see our world through the filter of "satisfied eyes," and for a moment, everything is good. We could even fall asleep very contentedly, reassuring ourselves that, "Yes, food is my comfort" (operant conditioning). Everything will be okay.

However, hours later, as you sit back to idly watch TV, your subconscious brings to your conscious mind what it had put aside hours before: all is not well. Not only that, it is the pits. Subtly, life's issues resurface that had been left on the back burner of your mind (e.g., the lack of intimacy in your life; bills to be paid; family obligations to meet; a job to go to; meetings to attend; and/or angry people to confront). Then, rather than to *sit-with-it*, you reach into the freezer for the ice cream you know is there, or into the pantry for a bag of chips, popcorn, doughnuts, or whatever snack food—once again telling yourself you are hungry.

You responded by heading for food—not wanting to deal with the uncomfortable thoughts. For this reason, I usually do not keep junk food in the house. I have even caught myself picking up a bag of chips in response to a sales ad, and because of *sitting-with-it* for so long I find I automatically ask myself, "Will I meet my goals eating this?" I usually put it back because I become aware of the rationalizations I am thinking to convince myself I need to make the purchase.

Too many times we choose to eat because to acknowledge we are bored, truly bored would be overwhelming. "What do you mean "I am bored? I have been working all day. I am tired. I deserve a break." If this sounds like you, I challenge you to choose not to eat while you pass the time away. What does it mean to you to relax? Watch TV? Watch a movie? Then watch it without food. No, I think it is more likely you are bored—bored because you know there is a lot to do and avoidance is your escape route. Then, you enroll others in this pastime and call it "family time," so it does not look or feel bad. You could also be eating to mask procrastination. After all, if I am sitting down with a bowl of popcorn watching my movie, after a long day at work, no one is going to remind me I had promised to fix the fence, mow the grass or write the novel I always said I was going to start.

And, it gets even better. I have heard clients say, "*I've found the more weight I gain, the less I'm approached for sex. I get to give it when I'm good and ready, not when the other expects it,*" and, "*No one is asking me to do chores around the house or help out, because they see how sick or uncomfortable I am with my back and knee pains.*" So now you get to be off the hook for a lot of things and whatever you do or contribute is appreciated. Who would not go for a set-up like this? Is this a familiar dialogue or scene for you? If so, recognize what it is costing you. The people in your world have made very special accommodations for you. It is time to stop taking and give back. It is time to carry your fair share of the load. Choose to make life better not only for those far away (e.g., contributing to your favorite charities), but choose to make life better for your loved ones right here.

Do not let your boredom mask your procrastination. Recognize that although you get to put off taking care of yourself, because you are feeling so overwhelmed, the cost is huge. Make a list of all the costs you currently incur because of your excess weight (ex. 30 extra pounds cost me *the ability to play with my kids,* etc.). List financial and non-financial costs and then choose to *sit-with-it.* Let the enormity of the costs sweep over you and choose differently. Do not get complacent—change cannot come from complacency.

Therefore, the challenge to *sit-with-it* is to enter the uncomfortable space and look at the thoughts and feelings to be dealt with. You have put off projects long enough; you have denied yourself the luxury bubble bath long enough; you have denied yourself the luxury of lighting those candles and sitting in their soft glow with soothing music or soft sounds long enough; you have denied your soul the rejuvenating exercise of meditation long enough; and you have denied yourself the opportunity to be pampered long enough. Question the thought, "I do not have time." Meet with yourself and ask your tender spirit what it needs, in the moment, to be fulfilled and satisfied. Honor yourself and your needs by listening and waiting for an answer. Remember, you are on a journey unlike any other you have been on before. Go through the process. Run to your healing. You are worth it!

We all know initially, everyone is all gung-ho to lose weight, "I can do this." And then something changes, something happens. A few weeks after the initial enthusiasm, I hear resignation in voices. I hear, "I can't do this," followed by giving up. In the past, I tried to drag some clients out of their *uncomfortableness* and get them to really look at their feeling of being uncomfortable. It was very challenging to try to shake some clients out of their resignation. Now, I remind them of their commitment—their goals—and they can usually identify they are just falling back into their old stories or old habits. Most are now able to lift themselves from their trance state. Because you see, the only one who can really wake you up is you. John Bradshaw sees this as one's "trance state," and it is very obvious this is what is going on. In other places, I have heard it referred to as your *story*. If I tried to break you out of your trance, you would miss doing the necessary work to prevent yourself from falling back into it—much like a butterfly needing to work its way out of its cocoon.

Sit-with-it requires that you remember your commitment: recall your planned coping strategies, and then follow through. *Sit-with-it* requires your ability to speak the truth to yourself. *Sit-with-it* throughout your day and do not wait until you are faced with temptation. Have your goals and commitment ever present before you. Do not forget you are *sitting-with* something. Use it to fend off nasty attitudes, road rage, mindless shopping sprees, unfruitful conversations, belligerence, indifference, hate or jealousy. When you *sit-with-it* you really get to be the person you want to be. It is not a one-time deal. It is continuous and it is a process. Commit to going through the process. Then, when your stomach rumbles after you have just eaten a meal, tell your stomach to s*it-with-it*.

Eventually, time will be your healer. Once you become engaged in the process, change will become easier. If you have stuck to your commitment to overall heath and wellness, it will become a habit to the point it is not a struggle. You will automatically begin to respond with healthier choices. I have clients tell me all the time, they can not believe the way they used to eat—once they have lost the weight. They are now successfully in the *maintenance stage*.

You will recognize you have reached the *maintenance stage* when you recognize your new healthy relationship with food is unlike anything you could have imagined in the past. You will feel and look better and will be committed to maintaining it. Begin . . . the rest gets easier.

Chapter 15

Feeling full

After many years of teaching weight loss, I am consistently faced with clients who want to "feel full" after I define what healthy eating looks like. It is true that the foods which make us feel full the fastest are usually high fat, pre-packaged, convenience foods. Take salads for example, volume-wise, unless a lot of extras (e.g. cheese, seeds, eggs, meat, high-fat salad dressings) are added, you may not "feel full" quickly enough and subsequently, will not feel satisfied—satiated. This chasing after being satisfied is another challenge to weight loss.

However, when you are overweight, you can no longer say you want to "feel full," because you have retrained your body to accept larger volumes. Instead you have to be content and satisfied with, "I just ate and it is enough." *Sit-with-it* as you move towards self-actualization.

Self-actualization can be described as *the need to be all that one can be* (Maslow's hierarchy of needs). Looking at this concept of arriving at a place where we feel we have reached our *fullest potential*. It is arguable to suggest that the struggle of losing weight is wrapped up in the idea, "if I am at the height of where I am supposed to be, why then am I not feeling satisfied?" If the goal is to be satisfied, this feeling of satisfaction is temporarily quenched when one feels "full." And subsequently, our overeating meets our self-actualizing needs. Thus, with this perception, weight loss is not achieved because no one wants to go around feeling unsatisfied, deprived or hungry.

In *sitting-with-it*, we recognize the feeling of being hungry is not a physiological one but a hunger associated with whatever need is not currently being met. Otherwise, we continue to think we are hungry and we *should* eat.

Understand that unmet needs are dynamic: changing, and will vary based on what you are actually thinking in response to an *A* event. This is another reason why journaling your emotions in response to eating is important. Get your journal and write down your emotional *ABC's*. In this instance, the *A* would be whatever situation you found yourself in (e.g., sitting at home alone). Your *B* could be: I should not be alone. I am hungry and should eat. Your *C* would be: to eat. But now, after practicing recognizing you *B*, you choose to change your *B* to: "I am hungry for attention but I do not need to eat for comfort. I choose to *scrapbook*" (pick something from the activity list you previously identified—refer to Chapter 4). What would the *C* (behavior and feeling) of this belief be? You would feel in control, happy and engaged.

You can see for yourself part of the answer to long-term weight loss and its maintenance will be in identifying what you are thinking. Your thoughts are directly linked to your feelings, and subsequently, the behaviors you exhibit.

To *sit-with-it*, means to stop and take the time to go through the RBT steps on a consistent basis until it becomes your new automatic response. Allow your stomach to shrink in size so smaller serving sizes will be "satisfying." Self-love is required to get to this stage and is possible. All too often people give in to the urge because the feeling of self-deprivation is such a strong and visceral feeling. Unfortunately, they turn to rationalizations and self-justifications, which take them away from their goals. They go to a negative place where they say, "I can't" and cut off any further progress.

How then can we get to the point where the stomach can return to its former, smaller self, and cut off shaming negative self-talk? *Sit-with-it.* There will be times when you resist telling yourself to *sit-with-it*, and you will avoid it so you can have what you want. However, when you tell yourself to *sit-with-it*, you will find it works and you will be able to avoid the temptation. Take the time to investigate when you choose to not *sit-with-it*, to help tease out your underlying belief as to why you continue to sabotage your own wellness goals. It may be a good idea to work with a therapist or counselor on an individual basis at this "stuck" place.

Also, to realize long-term weight maintenance means we have to remain in a dynamic process of awareness, so we can allow our bodies to get to this physiological state. Initially, getting to this state requires effort (e.g., planning life-style changes and behavior modifications—new and improved meal planning; changes in how food is prepared, stored, new shopping lists, restocking your pantry, and increased physical activity).

Part of remaining in this dynamic state to ensure the process continues, is to remain in a supportive setting once the goal has been attained at least on a monthly basis. You may need to be encouraged to continue in your new learned behavior. Without the behavior modifications and cognitive behavior changes, some may be unable to maintain momentum on their own and relapse. Again, I must emphasize the importance of working as a team with a physician, registered dietitian, counselor or therapist and/or support group.

You will find that *sitting-with-it* gives you access to other areas of your life (e.g., making a major purchase, going to a particular event or place or controlling your temper). Thus, eating represents only one of the ways in which we will not deprive ourselves. Add the temptation of easy credit card access—we are not used to putting things off—and you begin to see how the behaviors extend far beyond weight loss.

Another key to your maintenance goals is to engage those who are close to you. Share your new insights and understanding (if it is safe to do so). Be aware that these individuals may also be eating to fill an emotional void. If no one is available (or even if someone *is* available), continue to journal what you are experiencing. Many times our feelings go invalidated and we just set ourselves up for another inappropriate eating episode—*relapse.*

In *The Trusting Heart: Great News About Type A Behavior,* Redford Williams, M.D. writes, ". . . we must be realistic. Once a disease process has advanced beyond a certain point, the biology of the disease itself alters the situation and takes on a life of its own."

The urgency is here. The time is now. Do not wait for sickness and diseases to plague you before you get to the action stage. Start today to *sit-with-it* and go through the process to experience weight loss and its maintenance. How do I know you care? Because I have seen you in the emergency room after you have called 9-1-1. This tells me you want to live. Therefore, commit to a healthier lifestyle and honor the true you.

Chapter 16

What is the bottom line?

When you *sit-with-it*, what you are really *sitting with* is your commitment. For example, when I am committed to overall health and wellness, when I start to obsess about wanting a doughnut or getting the sweet treat or rewarding myself with food, I simply remind myself of my commitment to overall health and wellness. I choose to say, *sit-with-it*, which starts the process of *sitting-with-it*. Start to see it as a cat-and-mouse game:—we knowingly eat what we know we are supposed to avoid or we eat too much of something and then feel uncomfortable and guilty about having done it. Despite this, we continue to do the same thing again and again although some of us may gasp for air trying to get up a flight of three to six steps. But then, we make accommodations. What do we do? We try to avoid the steps altogether and take the elevator, or ramp, or just avoid places that have steps! It would seem we would just get so tired of it all, that we would want to see a change: see an improvement. But alas, this is not the case and more times than not, we just continue to add insult to injury, backache to our already beleaguered spine and more pressure and workload on our already over-exerted heart.

What is the purpose? What is the intent? What does it get us? Where do we end up? If one looks at life as a continuum, we step on and we eventually step off, where we do not know, but the cycle continues. Why don't we decide between now and the end, we will live the healthiest we can live, rather than just accept where we are? President Bill Clinton once said, "Don't give up when you lose. When you win, raise the bar."

Now, when you first think of eating, instead of saying, "I want that," or, "It would be nice to have that," change your thought to be "It would be nice to have this, however, I choose to sew (refer to your list) instead because I am committed to my weight loss goals."

Sitting-with-it means remembering your commitment on how you want to look after your goals are reached and then saying to yourself, "*Sit-with-it.*" In this case, replacing the craving is what you would have been committed to. The hardest part about *sit-with-it* is to say it. However, the more you practice saying and doing it, the easier it becomes and you would have effectively replaced the old habit of changing a want into a need. You would have changed the emotion of feeling deprived to one of being in control. To say, "*Sit-with-it*" when you are faced with situations where you previously would have given in to the temptation, now creates a space for making a rational choice.

Sit-with-it, in review

1) You have to *want* something different for yourself. You *must* want to change. It has to come from somewhere deep inside of you, where you give it your all. Your desire to be healthy must supersede everything else.
2) You have to *believe* change is necessary and vital.
3) You have to *be committed* to going through the steps.

When you sit with your commitment to go through the process, you will start to recognize how you do things. You can enter the madness and the chaos while maintaining control. You will deal with what needs to be dealt with and obtain your freedom from whatever it is you have been allowing control of your life.

Chapter 17

The Psycho-Social-Spiritual Connection

We are body, mind and soul. Body is our physical self, mind is our intellectual and emotional self and soul is the recognition there is a higher power than us—a creative force. For me the Higher Power is God, who came in the form of His Son Jesus Christ. Because of my mental/emotional, physical and soulful/spiritual wellness, I am now complete and whole. If at any time I do not feed each of my three parts, then I will not be whole and complete and will seek other ways to restore those parts to wellness. Sometimes it comes in the form of an addiction, among others, where some may look to drugs, sex, alcohol or food to heal an emotional emptiness rather than to acknowledge and express their feelings more appropriately.

You could be overeating your emotions. I have come to liken the challenge to weight loss to a love affair. Do you recall the movie "Doctor Zhivago," when Yuri and Lara first met up again and were standing in her living room? They looked at each other, knowing they were finally going to give in to sexual temptation and have an affair. You could feel the static energy between them, much like the energy generated when we obsess on food before we give in to the temptation of eating it. In this instance, I am talking about eating when you know you have already had enough, or you are overindulging.

You go through an eating frenzy where it is almost as though you do not know how to control yourself. You can't seem to get the food into you fast enough. This is where *sitting-with-it* calls to memory your commitment to being your word. Your word to being proactive and choosing an alternative. You gave your word to making an alternate choice or to pursue health and wellness, or to take better care of yourself. To *sit-with-it* requires your knowing you are going to relapse and to have a strategy in place for when those moments occur—so that it is not an "all or nothing day." Have a diversion ready to take the place of the obsessive thought and then do something else. For example, when Lara told Yuri his wife had visited her and left a letter for him. He must have felt really bad, just like we feel after we have broken our commitment. The story turns out to be a sad love story—a tragedy. Just like our lives will turn out to be tragic if we rescind our commitment to live a healthy lifestyle and take on the numerous illnesses we know will eventually occur. Again, reclaim your goal to a healthy lifestyle and *sit-with-it.*

As the days go by and you stay with your commitment to *sit-with-it* during times of temptation, you will become more aware of the excuses you give yourself for going forward with the behaviors. You will also recognize the many times you are not your commitment. Doing the work I do made me profoundly aware of the many times I told a lie—both to myself and to others, by rationalizing my inappropriate eating behaviors.

At first, you may start off by wanting something and then remember you are committed to weight loss. But then you may have it any way. The next time you begin to "want" something, have a conversation with yourself in which you remind yourself of the time you have invested in reaching your goal (you have probably tried multiple weight loss programs in the past), and *sit-with-it.* The next time you begin to "want" something, put into place the strategies you have already come up with (i.e., call a friend, journal or go for a walk).

Catharsis

Before you know it, you will be on your way as your self-talk reminds you tomorrow is another day and you can plan for it then. Each day will snowball into the next, and before you know it, you will feel this enormous pride of accomplishment riding on your back, reminding you: you can do this. As you journal, you will see the days of your commitment increase and you will want to go the extra mile. More strategies for coping will emerge. You will reward yourself with non-food items. You will begin to experience feelings you had previously submerged. Happy, healthy hormones will be released into your blood stream. You will heal from the inside-out and will be in a new place psychologically. Initially, others will not notice, but you will know and feel it on the inside. Soon, others will begin to wonder at the changes in you. They will not be able to pin-point it at first, because the change will first come in your attitude. Then as time goes by, they will see the visible signs as the pounds melt off. A certain glow will surround you and there will be lightness in your steps; an air of accomplishment will follow you. You will begin to experience people and situations differently. You may even find yourself in a meltdown, where you just break down and cry. Your tears may be of sorrow or joy, anger or elation, resentment or determination, fear or courage—and it will be okay. This is your time. Take the time to experience it.

Allow your body to unleash the many years of anguish you have kept bottled up. Allow yourself the release and the expression of self-love. You might even go for a drive or walk alone, just to try to sort it all out. But you will go through and you will get through. Whatever you do, do not allow yourself to run from your feelings. They are yours and they are valid. Embrace the new you. Embrace yourself in all your wonder, serenity and love. You are now more aware than you had ever thought possible. Your whole life has changed for the better and you are in the midst of it all. You are more beautiful, creative and vivacious. Applaud yourself! Dance for joy, or spend a quiet moment alone. Call up a loved one and share your journey. Share your new birth. Share the jewel you are. You have come full circle. You have started a journey that can only lead to more youthfulness, vitality and self-expression. You are in the process of arriving. You are feeling a lot more these days but you are also bouncing back with more resiliency than before. You may find yourself non-food shopping, redecorating or changing things around in your personal space. You will find you want the new you represented in a new and bolder way. Your bolder self will ask for what you want with both humility and pride. Not arrogant pride, but a pride borne out of your struggle to accomplish what you have accomplished. You are now well on your way to becoming the person you have longed to become.

Chapter 18

How long will this take? What's there to change?

They say it takes twenty-one days to reform a habit. For some, it may be sooner if they are convinced that what they are doing is long-term and not a temporary fix. To *sit-with-it* requires you recall being your commitment as well as to re-evaluating and refuting the self-defeating thoughts that yield landslides, failures and relapses on a daily basis.

I have helped many take the weight off and keep it off because of their commitment to healthy living and because of loving the new self that emerged. When you speak with these individuals, you do not hear regret and longing for a past way of living. There is no nostalgic longing after an illness laden life-style lost. They made a choice for health. When they *sit-with-it*, they enjoy healthy living rewards. Old unhealthy habits have been replaced with new and healthy automatic responses. This does not mean they are not tempted, but the tempting things have changed! They now see all their choices. They choose from a healthy menu of life's smorgasbord of choices. If all they were offered were healthy choices, they would find themselves navigating through familiar waters. They no longer feel *starved,* because their stomachs have shrunk to a smaller size. Before it took two servings to "feel full" and now only one serving is required to "feel full." This is partly why it is no longer a temptation.

They are looking through new lenses. They are *not* criticizing others for their choices because they understand and empathize because of where they have been. For me, a "recovering chocoholic," chocolate is no longer an issue. If I choose chocolate, it is because I choose it. I am no longer caught up in, "*I have to have chocolate.*"

I Can't = I can try, or I can too

Make it fun! For your purposes, change *I can't* to "I can try," or "I can too." No longer be willing to accept "I can't" to mean I cannot. It seems we have come to accept "I can't" as an excuse for being unable to control ourselves. However, I challenge you to see *I can't* as an abbreviation to "I can try" or "I can too." See *I won't* as "I will try," or "I will too."

Ask yourself . . .

In *The Best Question Ever,* author Andy Stanley recommends we ask ourselves before making a decision: "What is the wisest thing to do?" Phrased this way, if you are tempted by an extra serving or junk food, you can try to bring forth your prior goals and *sit-with-it.* This question caught my attention as I was on the stationary bike reading his book and thinking about the dessert I was going to treat myself with once I was finished with my workout. I asked myself, "What is the wisest thing to do?" and the floodgates opened a lot of alternatives which did not include dessert! It works. You just have to work it. The thought disappeared as I refuted the lies and reminded myself of the benefits I would reap by not giving in to the unhealthy choice. Instead, I meditated on how much healthier I would feel choosing a healthy alternative, especially after a workout! I was also able to recognize I was telling myself it was okay to have a dessert treat because of my hard workout. Yes, it would have been okay to eat a small slice of cake, but not immediately following a workout and not in a vulnerable moment. In other words, the rationalization I was making was erroneous (not the actual eating of the cake).

Define for yourself who YOU are and you will no longer be controlled by food. If you want to be helpless, then you will continue to turn to food. If you want to be who God made you to be, then food will not be an issue. You choose.

Choose to make a change for the future and to live a healthier and happier life, or stay where you are now in the past, and continue on the road to ill health. Again, you choose. I hope you will choose to make a change for the future on your unique journey to weight loss.

The truth behind weight loss and its maintenance is that it is possible following the *sit-with-it* process. Get ready, committed and convinced, and follow the steps. Once your weight loss goals have been realized, you will be able to stand in the *maintenance stage* of change. This is a good place to be. Understand relapses may occur, and it is okay to cycle back through the *preparation* and *action stage* of change. However, if you do not arrive at the *action* or *maintenance stage*, go back through this book, and allow yourself to really experience the process so you can achieve your weight loss goals. Go ahead. Start now. Find out first hand, how *sitting-with-it* becomes a habit that translates into weight loss, as you make healthy deposits into your wellness account.

Glossary of Terms

1. **Commitment**: Making a conscientious decision to follow through with a chosen plan, despite distractions.
2. **Being your word/commitment**: Doing what you say you are going to do.
3. **Our Stories**: our interpretations/perceptions of events that have occurred in our lives.
4. **Operant conditioning**: The theory that behavior can be controlled by rewards and punishments (termed by Edward L. Thorndike 1874-1949).
5. **Classical conditioning**: The theory that an event/outcome is paired to a behavior (seen with Pavlov's dogs—Ivan Pavlov (1849-1936)).

Author's Note

As an adjunct to this book, I strongly recommend you read the following books: *You and Your Emotions* by Maxie C. Maultsby, Jr., M.D. and Allie Hendricks, M.A.; *Healing the Shame That Binds You* and *Home Coming: Reclaiming and Championing Your Inner Child* by John Bradshaw, so as you go through the exercises presented in this book you will further your growth and get to a place where it is not a matter of being motivated, determined or disciplined, but rather a matter of being in a space of awareness where you choose. You will then know and believe you have a choice.

To help my clients manage the nutritious component of the *sit-with-it* concept, we use the Tri-Part-U® wellness solution meal plan where there are no forbidden foods, only variety—in their appropriate serving sizes—to promote optimum health and wellness. It focuses on the complete you. (For more information, visit www.tripartu.com).

To get on our mailing list, purchase the Tri-Part-U® meal plan, purchase an autographed copy of my book, schedule a private consultation or join our weight loss support group class, please write me: Anders Grant, Post Office Box 1390, Owings Mills, MD 21117, or visit the *www.tripartu.com* website, or email me: anders@tripartu.com.

References

American Dietetic Association. (1997). *RD Fact Sheet.* Retrieved October 12, 2006, from www.eatright.org/cps/rde/xchg/ada/hs.xsl/CADE_748_ENU_Print.htm

Barnhart, C.L. (Ed.). (1963). The American College Dictionary. New York: Random House.

Bradshaw, J. (1988). *Healing the Shame That Binds You.* New York: Bantam.

Bradshaw, J. (1990). *Home Coming: Reclaiming and Championing Your Inner Child.*

Clinical Guidelines on the Identification, Evaluation, and Treatment of Overweight and Obesity in Adults. (1998). Bethesda, MD: National Institutes, Health, National Heart, Lung, Blood Institute.

Clinton, B.(US President). (2005, October 26). US Senate Quorum Call. [Television broadcast].

Corey, G. (2000). *Theory & Practice of Group Counseling* (5th ed). Belmont, CA: Brooks/Cole.

Covey, S.R. (2004). *7 Habits of Highly Effective People.* New York: Free Press.

Griffen, A, Ponti, C. (Producers), Lean, D. (Producer/Director). Pasternak, B (Writer/Novel), Bolt, R. (Writer/Screen Play) 1965. Doctor Zhivago [Motion Picture]. United States: Metro-Goldwyn-Mayer (MGM) & Sostar S.A.

Hall, M., Curtis Chapman, S. (2003). Voice of Truth. On *Casting Crowns* [CD]. Nashville: Club Zoo Music/Peach Hill Songs 2/Sparrow Song/SWECS.

Holmes, D.S. (2001). *Abnormal Psychology* (4th ed). Needham, MA: Allyn & Bacon.

Holy Bible. (1988). Kings James Version. Nashville, TN: Holman Bible Publishers.

Konrad, C., Goode, C., Orent, K., Poster, M., Weinstein, B. & Weinstein H. (Producers), Rogers, S. (Writer) & Mangold, J. (Writer/Director). 2001. Kate & Leopold [Motion Picture]. United States: Konrad Pictures & Miramax Films.

Maultsby, M.C., Jr., M.D. (1990). *Rational Behavior Therapy.* Appleton, WI: Rational Self-Help Aids/I'ACT

Orman, Suze. (1999). *The Courage to be Rich.* New York: Riverhead Books.

Prochaska, J.O., DiClemente, C.C., & Norcross, J.C. (1992). In Search of How People Change, *American Psychology.* 47(9), 1102-1114).

Schwartz, B. (2001). *I Run, Therefore I Am—NUTS!* Champaign, IL: Human Kinetics.

Sharf, R.S., (2002). *Applying Career Development Theory to Counseling* (3rd ed.). Brooks/Cole.

Stanley, A. (2004). The Best Question Ever. Sisters, Oregon: Multnomah Publishers.

Thoele, S.P. (1996). *Heart Centered Marriage, Fulfilling Our Natural Desire for Sacred Partnership.* Berkley, CA.: Conari Press.

Williams, R., M.D. (1989). *The Trusting Heart: Great News About Type A Behavior.* New York: Times Books.

Suggested Readings

Bradshaw, John. (1988). *Healing the Shame That Binds You.* New York: Bantam.

Bradshaw, John. (1992). *Creating Love, the Next Great Stage of Growth.* New York: Bantam Books.

Bradshaw, John. (1990). *Home Coming: Reclaiming and Championing Your Inner Child.*

Maultsby, M.C., Jr., M.D. & Hendricks, A. (1974). *You and Your Emotions.* Lexington, KY: Rational self-Help Books.

Orman, Suze, (1997). *The 9 Steps to Financial Freedom.* New York: Crown Publishers, Inc.

Orman, Suze. (1999). *The Courage to be Rich.* New York: Riverhead Books.

Resources

Landmark Education Seminar: *www.landmarkeducation.com*
To find a registered dietitian near you, visit: *www.eatright.org*

About the Author

Anders Grant is a licensed and registered dietitian. She earned a Baccalaureate degree in Foods and Nutrition from the State University of California in Pomona. Later, she interned at North Carolina State University in the field of dietetics and sat for her state board exam. Subsequent to that, she earned a Masters degree in counseling education from McDaniel College in Westminster Maryland. Anders Grant has been a nutritionist for the past fourteen years. For the past four years, she has worked in the field of clinical dietetics with specialties in weight loss and eating disorders. She is passionate about her work and the friendships that have resulted. Anders has a deep love for the sport of running, regularly running marathons and ultra-marathons. Anders has three children who bring joy and delight to her life and are responsible for the balance she brings to her profession as a nutrition and wellness expert.